Gerontological Social Work Practice in the Community

The *Journal of Gerontological Social Work* series:

• *Gerontological Social Work Practice in Long-Term Care*, edited by George S. Getzel and M. Joanna Mellor

• *A Healthy Old Age: A Sourcebook for Health Promotion with Older Adults (Revised Edition)*, by Stephanie FallCreek and Molly Mettler

• *The Uses of Reminiscence: New Ways of Working with Older Adults*, edited by Marc Kaminsky

• *Gerontological Social Work in Home Health Care*, edited by Rose Dobrof

• *Gerontological Social Work Practice in the Community*, edited by George S. Getzel and M. Joanna Mellor

• *Social Work and Alzheimer's Disease*, edited by Rose Dobrof

Gerontological Social Work Practice in the Community

George S. Getzel
M. Joanna Mellor
Editors

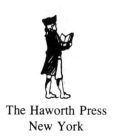

The Haworth Press
New York

Gerontological Social Work Practice in the Community has also been published as *Journal of Gerontological Social Work,* Volume 8, Numbers 3/4, Spring/Summer 1985.

The Haworth Press, Inc., 28 East 22 Street, New York, NY 10010

Library of Congress Cataloging in Publication Data
Main entry under title:

Gerontological social work practice in the community.

   "Has also been published as Journal of gerontological social work, volume 8, no. 3/4, spring/summer 1985"—T.p. verso.
   Includes bibliographies and index.
   1. Social work with the aged—United States—Addresses, essays, lectures.
2. Community health services for the aged—United States—Addresses, essays, lectures. I. Getzel, George S. II. Mellor, M. Joanna. [DNLM: 1. Health Services for the Aged.
2. Social Work. W1 J0669NS v.8 no.3/4 / WT 30 G37676]
HV1461.G48 1985   362.6'042   85-2767.
ISBN 0-86656-145-5
ISBN 0-86656-256-7 (pbk.)

Gerontological Social Work Practice in the Community

Journal of Gerontological Social Work
Volume 8, Numbers 3/4

CONTENTS

SECTION IV: PERSPECTIVES FROM THE WORLD OF PRACTICE: EMERGING SOCIAL WORK APPROACHES AND SETTINGS

About the Editors

GEORGE S. GETZEL, DSW, is Professor at Hunter College School of Social Work, City University of New York, N.Y. As a consultant and author of several articles, Dr. Getzel's interests include group work, social work with the aged and research in value dilemmas in working with the elderly, as well as assistance to crime victims and special at risk populations. Dr. Getzel is a Fellow of the Gerontological Society of America, member of several editorial boards and consultant to social agencies and national organizations.

M. JOANNA MELLOR, MS, is Assistant Project Director with the Third Age Center, Fordham University, N.Y. and formerly Program Analyst with the Natural Supports Program, Community Service Society, N.Y. Her interests include the relationship of social work research to practice, the informal support system of the frail elderly and the development of self-help and client advocacy groups. As co-director of Network Associates, Ms. Mellor is a consultant and trainer in the above areas and is author of several articles.

RENEE SOLOMON, DSW, *Associate Professor, Columbia University School of Social Work, NY, NY*
SHELDON TOBIN, PhD, *Director, Ringel Institute of Gerontology, Albany, NY*
TERESA JORDAN TUZIL, MSW, *Consultant on Aging, New York, NY*
EDNA WASSER, MSW, *Consultant, Fellow, Gerontological Society, Miami, FL*
MARY WYLIE, PhD, *Professor, Department of Social Work, University of Wisconsin, Madison, WI*

Contributors

ROGER BAKER, MSW, formerly Program Developer and Analyst at the Community Service Society, N.Y., is now a Computer Programmer. Social work interests include housing and community services for the aged as related to long term care needs.

SONDRA M. BRANDLER, DSW, is a Founder and past Executive Director of the Jay Senior Center in Brooklyn, New York. In addition to aging families, Ms. Brandler's professional interests include the use of poetry with older persons. She is author of "Poetry, Group work and the Aged," *Journal of Gerontological Social Work,* 1979.

DAVID FELDSTEIN, MSW, is Assistant Borough Director, Bronx, N.Y. Jewish Association for Services for the Aged and Adjunct Associate Professor at the Hunter School of Social Work, City University of New York, N.Y. Mr. Feldstein's interests include long range planning and the intersection of social policy and technology. He is co-author of *Preventing Chronic Dependency,* Community Service Society, N.Y., 1970.

HARRIET GOODMAN, MSW, is Research Associate for Supportive Care Services at New York Hospital, N.Y., and was previously Senior Social Worker/Supervisor of the Group Work Department at the Jewish Guild for the Blind, N.Y. In addition to social work services for the blind elderly, Ms. Goodman's professional interests focus on terminal care.

SUSAN GUTWILL, MSW, co-developed and implemented a social service program for the New Jersey District Council 65, United Automobile Workers. As a union social worker, her interests include industrial social work, special counseling, self-help groups and program needs of the working class. Ms. Gutwill is currently in private practice, specializing in compulsive eating disorders.

MIRIAM HABIB, MSW, is Director of the Morris County Family Mediation and Conciliation Services. Developer of social service programs for New Jersey District Council 65 Ms. Habib has special interest in training and developing a network of natural helpers at the work site. She is author of several papers including "Working in a Labor Union to reach retirees," *Social Casework,* March, 1980.

MARGARET E. HARTFORD, PhD, is Professor Emerita of Gerontology and Social Work at the School of Gerontology and the School of Social Work, University of Southern California. First Director of the Leonard Davis School of Gerontology at the U.S.C., Dr. Hartford is an educator and consultant. Her interests include curriculum development, group work and retirement planning. Dr. Hartford has published numerous articles, is author of *Groups on Social Work,* Columbia University Press and is currently preparing *Working with and on behalf of Older adults in the Human Services. Applied Gerontology,* Columbia University Press.

MARC KAMINSKY, MSW is co-director of the Institute on Humanities, Art and Aging of the Brookdale Center on Aging, Hunter College, City University of New York, N.Y. Author of several papers, Mr. Kaminsky is a leading proponent of the arts by, for and with the aging. Books include *What's Inside You. It Shines Out of You.* N.Y. Horizon Press, 1974 and four books of poems published by the University of Illinois Press, including *Daily Bread* and *Table with People,* 1982.

CHARLOTTE KIRSCHNER, DSW, is Director of Geriatric Family Service, New York City, providing comprehensive services to families and their frail elderly. Her interests include the role of the social worker in home care, family counseling and pre-planning and family crisis intervention. Dr. Kirschner is author of numerous articles.

HARRY R. MOODY, PhD, is the Director of the National Policy Center on Education, Leisure and Continuing Opportunities at the National Council on Aging, Washington, D.C. Dr. Moody is co-editor of the Human Values and Aging Newsletter and Adjunct Associate Professor of Philosophy at Hunter College, City University of New York. His interests include the ethical dilemmas in gerontology.

MARIA ROSENBLOOM, MSW, is Assistant Professor at the Hunter College School of Social Work, City University of New York, where she teaches clinical social work practice. A survivor of the Holocaust, she has extensive experience relevant to the impact of genocide on survivors and their families. Author of "Implications of the Holocaust for Social Work," *Social Casework,* April 1983.

HARRIET RZETELNY, MSW, is on the staff of the Brookdale Center on Aging of Hunter College, City University of New York. Ms. Rzetelny is involved in training staff of senior centers, nursing homes and other related aging facilities. Her special interests are in the problems and stresses of aging. She is author of "Working with Frail Elderly in Senior Centers" prepared for the New York State Human Resources Administration, D.S.S.

ROBERT SALMON, DSW, is Associate Dean and Professor of Social Work at Hunter College School of Social Work, City University of New York. In addition to gerontology, Dr. Salmon's interests include group work, administration and supervision within the social work profession and drug use and abuse. He is the author of numerous articles.

GARY B. SELTZER, PhD, is Assistant Professor of Community Health and Family Medicine, Brown University and Study Director and Clinical Psychologist at Memorial Hospital, Pawtucket, Rhode Island. Interests include study of the impact of institutionalization on retarded adults, community residences and functional assessment in primary care. Dr. Seltzer is co-author of *Context for Competence: A study of Retarded adults living and working in the Community,* Cambridge Educational Projects, Inc. and a regular contributor to professional journals.

MARSHA MAILICK SELTZER, PhD, is Assistant Professor at Boston University School of Social Work (Research) and also Assistant Professor within the Sociology Department. As consultant and director of evaluation for a variety of programs, Dr. Seltzer's interests lie in the area of community care and housing for the mentally retarded. She is the author of numerous papers and published articles.

CYNTHIA STUEN, MSW, is Director of Community Education at Brookdale Institute on Aging and Adult Human Development, Columbia University, and Associate Research Scientist, Columbia University School of Social Work. Interested in older adult learning and voluntarism with University faculty retirees, Ms. Stuen is author of several articles and of the manual "Seniors teaching seniors. A manual for training older adult teachers," Brookdale Institute.

DAVID SUMBERG, MSW, is Senior Social Worker of St. Lukes Hospital Comprehensive Alcoholism Training Program. He is a specialist in individual and group psychotherapy in which he has a private practice and is currently writing a book on the subject of Group therapy with Alcoholics. Mr. Sumberg is also author of *Checklists—88 Essential Lists to Help You Organize Your Life,* Crown Publishers, 1982.

ELIZABETH ZBOROWSKY, MSSA, is Research Assistant at Case Western Reserve University, School of Applied Sciences and formerly the Assistant Director of Social Work at the Benjamin Rose Institute, Cleveland. In addition to her interests in protective services for the elderly, Ms. Zborowsky has researched and published articles (under the name Elizabeth Kerns) on the subject of short term treatment for adolescents.

Foreword

This is the second volume in our Social Work Practice Series, edited by George S. Getzel and M. Joanna Mellor, and published by The Haworth Press. The first volume, *Gerontological Social Work Practice in Long-Term Care,* was published in 1982.

In this new volume, as its title indicates, the authors have turned to the nature of practice with older people in the community. The range and variety of subjects addressed by the authors testify to the complexities which confront social workers, and other helping professions, in their work with older people. Several of the articles in this volume call our attention to subgroups within the older population, who merit special concern: Elizabeth Zborowsky reports on a protective services research-demonstration program conducted at the Benjamin Rose Institute in Cleveland, and concludes her article with a definition of four issues which must be addressed in the development of protective services for older people.

Seltzer and Seltzer write about the elderly mentally retarded. They argue that the increase in the life span of developmentally disabled persons means that the aged cohort in the United States is including a steadily growing subgroup of the mentally retarded, and that little attention has been paid to this group in either the field of mental retardation or gerontology. This is a "State of the Art" article, including a brief, but very useful "definition of the population" which provides a framework for readers who are not familiar with the field of mental retardation; and analysis of the demographics of this subgroup, and of particular utility for workers in the aging network, a discussion of the special problems of the elderly mentally retarded.

Of the same genre are Feldstein's piece on the chronic mentally frail; Goodman's on the elderly blind; Sumburg's on elderly alcoholics; and Rosenbloom's on Holocaust survivors in later life. All of these articles reinforce the necessity for workers to understand the heterogeneity of the older cohort, and each provides the reader with knowledge about the characteristics and special service needs of a particular subgroup.

Brandler's article on the Senior Center and the Habib and Gutwill piece on the union setting both look at aspects of social work practice in these two settings, and Kirschner delineates a systems approach to work with the families of older people. The article by Kaminsky represents a further development of his work on writing and reminiscing in old age, and Salmon contributes a piece which combines theory and practice in an analysis of work with older volunteers. Rzetelny, deals with four losses which characterize the later years of many, and which are the source of the emotional stress which social workers see in many of their clients; and Stuen contributes a useful summation of outreach services to older people.

The first three chapters constitute a theoretical framework for the book: Getzel begins with a presentation of eight "Themes" which he says "represent major issues" for social workers in the field of gerontology. Moody argues in his "Critical Perspective for Policy and Action" that ". . . a pervasive ideology has grown up in our society around old age. . . (which) . . . express(es) a dominant ideology of old age that itself contributes to the problem of aging in America." All readers may not agree with Moody's position, but none of us is free to ignore the argument he presents. The final work in this theoretical framework is that by Hartford on normative growth and development in the later years.

We present this volume with pride and with certainty that workers in the field will find it a useful collection, and one which helps them understand the needs of special populations of older people, the nature of practice in the community, and some of the policy and practice issues which they confront in their work.

Rose Dobrof

Gerontological
Social Work Practice
in the Community

Section I

MAKING SENSE
OF GERONTOLOGICAL PRACTICE
IN THE 1980s

Chapter I

Critical Themes
for Gerontological Social Work Practice

George S. Getzel

What is gerontological social work? This chapter will look at the special skills demanded of social workers who engage in work with an aging population. An understanding of gerontological social work practice emerges from the moment-to-moment, day-to-day encounters between the professionals and their aging clients.

Central to this analysis is a working definition of skill. Virginia Robinson writes that skill is "the capacity to set in motion and control a process of change in a specific material in such a way that the change that takes place in the material is effected with the greatest consideration for and utilization of the quality and capacity of the material."[1] Implied in this definition is the intertwined process of thinking, feeling and acting that are elicited by the worker's contact with old people in their social context.

Skill is linked to the systemizing rigor of practice theory that responds to the particulars of older peoples' lives. William Schwartz, a seminal thinker on the nature of skill and its relationship to practice theory, notes the circular nature of action and practice theory. He writes,

> For a theory of practice is a theory of action, and action is not deductible from either knowledge or intention working alone. If we know everything there is to know, we would still have to decide what to do; and if purposes were impeccable, the action based on them would still not be self-evident. Each of these areas influence and limit each others' in every specific situation; given the appropriate evidence, and given a set of valued outcomes, the principles of action provide the implementing force.[2]

Skills, therefore, are conditioned by what the worker knows, values and does. Practical theory is grounded on the undulating flow of events of social living. The changing world of the older person creates special opportunities and constraints on the social worker's ability to be helpful. A social worker with a serious commitment to serve the aging must persist in updating his or her knowledge about the nature of the aging process and the implications of the environment for the older person's growth, health and social integration.

The gerontological social worker faces perennial problems in the course of service. I will identify some of these problems and the underlying issues of knowledge, intent and action that surround the demands of practice. This selective view of practice problems will, I hope, strike a responsive chord in those workers who are engaged daily in addressing the pressing needs of older persons. As we witness the plight of the aging, the need for action may preclude careful and extended reflection of the overarching dimensions of problems, thereby limiting alternative modes of intervention. The gerontological social worker may feel, with considerable justification, that there is a chasm between the reality of aging and the ready knowledge available to deal with practice concerns.

Berger and Luckmann make a useful distinction between the concept of social reality—"a quality appertaining to phenomena that we recognize as having a being independent of her own volition" and knowledge "the certainty that phenomena are real and they possess specific characteristics."[3] The persistent tensions between the reality of practice with and for the aging and the social worker's knowledge of practice often creates disequilibrating effects on the serious practitioner. In the face of tensions and uncertainty, the worker may find it tempting to make global or extravagant claims of skill—"I know about the elderly because people are people." This innocent homespun rationalization is used by the well-intentioned social worker as a protection against upsetting reactions toward older persons and their situation. If there is to be a dynamic field of gerontological social work, practitioners must permit and for that matter encourage the close examination of the problems arising out of work with older people in order to peel away a naive, indulgent view of the aging as curious oddities or aversive objects. Only then can social workers acquire differentiated assessments of older persons. To this end, core practice themes will be identified and discussed. Themes arise out of the efforts of social workers to apprehend the needs of the elderly and to engage them as fully as possible in the helping process. An understanding of these themes influences the skills and interventive strategies and methods.

CORE THEMES FOR PRACTICE

The following themes represent major issues for social work practice *with* and *for* the aged.

Theme 1—The Paradox of Personality and Aging

Gordon Allport writes that "Personality is less a finished product than a transitive process. While it has some stable features, it is at the same time continuously undergoing change. The first fact that strikes us is the uniqueness of both the process and the product."[4] Does this description of human personality obtain for older persons? Hesitantly we may say yes. Behind our pause lie doubts about the stability of personality against the corrosive disease-like effects of the aging process. In short, we look twice to see if an old person is "all there" whenever change is detected in his or her cognitive and emotional functioning. A social worker may see aging as precluding older persons' abilities to meet new challenges in the environment. Sometimes frightening losses in physiological functioning blind workers to evidences of adaptation and growth.

Old persons themselves toil with acceptance of personal aging. Rosow suggests the elderly avoid age identification in response to negative societal valuations.[5] It is not unusual for a person sixty-five years or older to call themselves middle age or prefer euphemistic age labels, "senior citizen" or "retired person," than the designation "aged" or "elderly."[6] They may also wish to associate with different aged groups and paradoxically associate with persons very close to their age.[7] Inclusion of old age into one's self-concept is a complicated and highly variable process. For that matter is it easy for a champion long-distance runner to accept a "competitive life" that ends at the age thirty? Can the runner then be reconciled to running with a group of superannuated joggers his own age?

To view aging and human personality together requires that social workers make finely honed judgments about an older person's drives, needs, perceptions, valuations and capacities. Biology insinuates itself deeply in the assessment task of gerontological social workers. Old people may become hostage to organ weakness. We watch them with an underlying dread.

Ernest Becker sees the clash between personality and biology as "an existential paradox" called, "The condition of individuality within finitude." He writes

> a human being is out of nature and hopelessly in it; he is dual, up in the stars and yet housed in a heart-pumping, breath-gasp-ing body. . . Man is literally split in two: he has an awareness of his uniqueness in that he sticks out of nature with a towering majesty, and yet he goes back into the ground a few feet in order to blindly dumbly rot and disappear forever.[8]

Thus the challenges of living, for the old, is to search for meaning and to encounter heroically the limits of time.

A social worker must learn to discern the variety of personality styles among the old facing similar and common life tasks. A social worker's intellectual preparation often precedes emotional integration of these painful recognitions from practice.

Theme 2—Aging as Loss and Adaptation

Closely related to the previous theme is the recognition of loss and adaptation as a normative event and process respectively. Butler and Lewis describe loss as the predominate emotional theme of aging. Losses of spouses, friends, health, social status and economic security are likely occurrences for many.[9] How do old persons cope with losses of people and situations which have conventionally defined their personhood? Direct practice constantly points to old people's resilience and ingenuity in handling loss. Social workers intervene when adaptive capacity is blocked or tasks are too difficult. Casework and group support programs are helpful approaches to handle the normative crises of aging. While there are no absolute substitutes for the loss of kin and friends, social supports may take the edge off the day-to-day dislocations of widowhood and other losses. Social workers must have the abilities to develop and to deliver these services. This requires an understanding of interventive sequencing with the specific crises of late life.

Theme 3—Dependence and Environment

To grow more fully human is to acknowledge the differentiated human personality and its interdependencies which provide support and foster growth and change.

As an older person's physiological capacities decrease, their vulnerability to the environment increases. Powell Lawton writes,

> In a real sense the individual's 'personality' must be defined partly in terms of the context in which it appears. A positive supporting environment will allow the continuation of competent behavior and the positive inner experience of competence while the behavior limited environment will foster a loss of competence.[10]

The integrity of personality is sustained by the goodness of fit between the older person and the environment which includes physical and interpersonal space, access to services and to other enriched environments.

The social workers' assessment of needs and their subsequent interventions must embody an understanding that the environment affects the physical and emotional well-being of the elderly. A social worker's skill in environmental manipulation for the impaired elderly may provide a degree of mobility and independence that has enormous meaning for older persons. Advocacy in this area is a very significant social work role.

Theme 4—Care and Caring as Virtues

Abraham Joshua Heschel, the religious philosopher in a talk before physicians reminded them that the word cure originates from the word care which is related to caras or heart. He stated that, "The truth of being human is gratitude. The secret of existence is appreciation, its significance is revealed in reciprocity. Mankind will not die for lack of information; it may perish for lack of appreciation."[11]

Like physicians, social workers search out beneficial treatments that will relieve suffering by removing the causes of misery. The magic bullet often eludes us. We meet the aged who embody the existential paradox. Ivan Illich suggests that we rethink our medicalized ideas of health and accept the limits of science and medicine. He writes that, "Man's consciously lived fragility, individuality and relatedness makes the experience of pain, of sickness and death an integral part of life."[12]

As old people face the limits of time and the tragedies of existence—death, illness and meaninglessness—social workers discover the limits of action. Social workers often need help with the ministering role of being there, bearing witness and on occasion, assisting older persons to search for meaning at the brink of the unknown or nothingness. In short, care and caring are virtues.

Theme 5—Age Grading and Relationship

The helping relationship is often a meeting between young and old, and it is not without its problems. Age distinctions are taught to us from early age. With age comes opportunities, sanctions and responsibilities.[13] The interpersonally reinforced grading of human beings according to age must be understood and used in the helping process. Old persons express powerful emotions to young workers, not only for what they symbolize from the past, dead or dissolute children and lost lovers, but as representatives of the present and of a future denied to them.

Social workers and old people must together accept the realization that intergenerational contacts are characterized by mutual unknown-ness and powerful emotions. Exploration of each party's relational assumptions is a necessary part of working together. Young workers have much to learn about the unique historic experiences of the elderly and the elderly must come to terms with aspects of their aging through exploring the meaning of being helped by the young.

Theme 6—Intergenerational Reciprocity

The flow of mutual aid between generations, through the systems of kin, friends and neighbors and the aged is repeatedly documented in the social gerontology. The myth of the isolated elderly abandoned by their kin and the community is widely held by social workers despite findings that most older persons have children who live nearby and frequently visit. Families, friends and neighbors are the most significant source of aid to community aged as they become less able to function independently. Informal social supports are continuous sources of social contact, material aid and instrumental assistance. Old persons are, in turn, significant sources of aid to their children and to others. Even older persons without available kin are apt to have neighbors as social supports.[13] Some studies indicate that even when older persons have had troubled relations with their children, mutuality is maintained into the late life.

Social workers have challenging roles in assisting kin and others maintain their caregiving function. Middle aged children and elderly spouses may be overwhelmed by the emotional, physical and familial stresses surrounding caregiving responsibilities.[14] Family members frequently are distressed by decisions that they must make. Competing generational claims, and the need for respite and other supportive services will grow as the proportion of very old persons and functionally impaired aged increase. Social workers have a significant role in interpreting the effects of aging on family life.[15] Innovative approaches in providing episodic and continuing support and assistance to families and other informal service providers are new important areas of practice skill and program development. Service to elderly is inseparable from activities done on their behalf by kin and community supports.

Theme 7—Corrective Action in an Ageist Society

An advocacy perspective remains a major focus of gerontological social work. Age stratification and age grading are part of social institutions. While the old must make way for the young, flagrant indifference and prejudices towards the elderly by formal organizations are too frequent. Institutional and cultural abuses of the elderly require that social workers be knowledgeable about rights to life sustaining income, health, housing and other benefits and entitlements. The popular culture must be questioned when it limits older person's opportunities and personal freedom. Skill in and commitment to case, class and professional advocacy strategies become especially significant as resources are diminished in this period of reaction. The budget may not get a chance to gray, before the young and old confront each other for limited social welfare dollars.

Theme 8—Transcendence and Creativity

One of the most exciting aspects of working with the elderly occurs as social workers experience older persons creative expressions in the face of bodily decline and the prospect of death. Becker says, "What man really fears is not so much extinction, but extinction with *insignificance.* Man wants to know his life has somehow counted if not for himself, then at least in a larger scheme of things, that is, has left a trace, a trace that has meaning."[16]

Awareness of death is part of old age. Otto Rank and others have suggested that it is a prime motive in all human beings regardless of age.[17] Robert Butler in his classic paper on reminiscence writes that the awareness of death prompts the aging person to go through an active process of "life review"—searching for personal serenity by coming to terms with the loose threads of historic past conflicts carried into late life.[18]

Jung identifies reminiscence as a response associated with old age. The aged may benefit from actively reflecting on past memories and the symbolism behind images of the past. Jung in his autobiography *Memories, Dreams, Reflections* gives personal form to this pursuit.[19] Another persuasive example of active engagement of past images and the stress of old age can be found in Florida Scott-Maxwell's *The Measure of My Days.*[20]

Reminiscence as social interaction links the older generations with young ones. At times old persons amuse themselves and others with elaborated and embroidered recollections. The issues of the present are translated into reminiscences that may ease adjustment to the serial losses of old age, confirming the constancy of self-concept and enhancing self-esteem.

Meyerhoff believes that in old age "life reviewing" creates deepened and enlarged ideas about our identities, "personal myths" that sustain us and contribute to the well-being of peers and progeny.[21] Butler also emphasizes the potential for the elderly to create new images of themselves. Butler indicates that many of the choices we make in life are "enforced" and do not reflect our secret "parallel infra-life."[22] Death hones our visions of life by opening the repressions of lost opportunities.

Old people can benefit from our willingness to hear their recollections, poems and autobiographical statements. If we are truly able to listen to them, the boundaries which separate us will dissolve into mutual benefit. First, the practitioner must confront the natural dread implicit in older person's intimations of mortality. Then, older persons will find a concrete connection to pass down their personality bounded efforts to maintain constancy and continuity with the world that remains before and after they are gone. Their efforts, however faltering or failed they may be, speak to the persistence and indomitability of human life even in the face of the inescapable.

CONCLUSION

The demands of each practice theme appear awesome in their complexity and emotional consequences for the gerontological social worker. Only through the emerging specializations in aging in social work curriculums on the master's level and structured continuing education, can practitioners develop creative programs and demonstrate those skills to meet the current and emerging needs of older persons in the community. Amidst the fads and fashions of our day which often betray social purposes and informed compassion, social workers must demonstrate, through their skills, an articulate concern for the aged.

REFERENCES

1. Virginia P. Robinson, "The Meaning of Skill," *Training for Skill in Social Casework*, Philadelphia: University of Pennsylvania Press, 1942, pp. 11-12.
2. William Schwarz, "Between Client and System: Mediating Function," in Robert W. Northen and Helen Northen (Eds.), *Theories of Social Work With Groups*, New York: Columbia University Press, 1976, p. 182.
3. Peter L. Berger and Thomas Luckmann, *The Social Construction of Reality*, Garden City, N.Y., Anchor Books, 1967, p. 1.
4. Gordon W. Allport, *Becoming: Basic Consideration for a Psychology of Personality*, New Haven: Yale University Press, 1955, p. 19.
5. Rosow, Irving, *The Social Integration of the Aged*, New York: Free Press, 1967.
6. Daum, Menachem, "Preferences for Age-Mixed Social Integration," in *Age or Need?* Bernice L. Neugarten, Beverly Hills, CA: Sage Publications, 1982, pp. 247-262.
7. Ibid.
8. Becker, Ernest, *The Denial of Death*, New York: Free Press, 1973, pp. 26-27.
9. Butler, Robert N. and Myrna Lewis, *Aging and Mental Health*, St. Louis, C. V. Mosby, 1977, p. 36.
10. Lawton, M. Powell, "Psychology of Aging" in William C. Bier (Ed.), New York: Fordham University Press, 1974, p. 81.
11. Heschel, Abraham Joshua, *The Insecurity of Freedom*, New York: Schocken, 1972, p. 26.
12. Illich, Ivan, *The Medical Nemesis*, New York: Bantam Books, 1976, p. 272.
13. Riley, Matilda White and others, *Aging and Society, Vol. III A Sociology of Age Stratification*, New York: Russell Sage Foundation, 1972.
14. Shanas, Ethel, "The Family as a Social Support System in Old Age," *Gerontologist*, 19, April 1979, pp. 144-169, Cantor, Marjorie, "Life Space and the Social Support System of Inner City Elderly of New York," *Gerontologist*, 15, February 1975, pp. 23-34 and Sussman, Marvin and Lee Burchinal, "Kin Family Network: Unheralded Structure in Current Conceptualization of Family Functioning," *Marriage and Family Living*, 24, August 1962, pp. 231-240.
15. Getzel, George S., "Social Work with Family Caregivers to the Aged," *Social Casework*, Vol. 62, April 1981, pp. 201-209, Getzel, George S. "Group Work with Kin and Friends Caring for the Elderly," *Social Work With Groups*, Vol. 5, No. 2, pp. 91-102, and Silverstone, Barbara and Helen K. Hyman, *You and Your Aging Parents* New York: Pantheon Press, 1976.
16. Becker, Ernest, *Escape From Evil*, New York: Free Press, 1975, p. 4.
17. See Rank, Otto, *Art and Artist: Creative Urge and Personality Development* New York: Agathon Press, 1968 and Becker, Ernest, *Escape from Evil*.
18. Butler, Robert N., "The Life Review: An Interpretation of Reminiscence in the Aged," *Psychiatry*, 126, 1963, pp. 65-76.

19. Jung, Carl G., *Memories, Dreams, Reflections*, New York: Vintage, 1961.
20. Scott-Maxwell, Florida, *The Measure of My Days*, New York: Dutton, 1979.
21. Meyerhoff, Barbara, *Number Our Days*, New York: Dutton, 1979.
22. Butler, Robert N., "Look Forward to What?," *American Behavioral Scientist*, 14, September-October, 1970, pp. 121-128.

Chapter II

A Critical Perspective for Policy and Action

Harry R. Moody

My argument in this paper is that a pervasive ideology has grown up in our society around old age. In using the term "ideology" and not a more familiar term like "stereotype" or "myth," I am deliberately taking up a position quite different from how gerontology has typically approached the problem of falsely held images about old age.[1] The prevalence of such falsely held images is beyond dispute: Americans in general, and old people themselves too, hold a dismal picture of what aging in America is like.[2] Gerontologists typically deplore such misinformation and call for more public education to dispel the negative image of old age. Advocates for the elderly seek to challenge patterns of discrimination under the category of "ageism." But amid this high-minded attack on false images, an important question remains unexamined. Why do these false images—these "stereotypes" and "myths"—persist?[3] What motivates their persistence and whose interest do they serve?

My point here is to underscore that the images that prevail are not lamentable mistakes or fears easily correctable by public education. My claim is more far-reaching. These distortions express a dominant ideology of old age that itself contributes to the problem of aging in America. Those who work as advocates on behalf of the aging are themselves deeply affected by distortions of perspective. Even the enterprise of academic gerontology is not immune from these distortions. What presents itself as "impartial" academic inquiry is often very far from that. The academic discipline of gerontology is distorted by a failure to examine competing paradigms that might lead to very different directions for theory and practice.[4] Among social scientists, as well as practitioners, values and assumptions

13

about old age are contaminated by the distorting power of ideology. Those distortions seriously compromise the effectiveness of advocacy, of scientific research, and of public policy.

Finally, the most insidious element of the current ideology of old age is that it is not recognized as such. Within the boundaries of that competition of ideas, we entertain the appearance of an "objective" or "rational" view of society: apparently the very opposite of an official ideology. But the distorting power of ideological thinking reaches its triumph by persuading us that ideology has ceased to exist. A more accurate way of putting the matter would be to say that the power of ideology in our society has become invisible:

> Today our ideologies are disguised. Their language has changed. The utopian element has disappeared. One might say that our own society holds some vague belief in democratic progress through the application of science to human affairs and that in recent times this belief has come to include social science. The special application of science in social affairs represents our commitment to the rational improvement of our society. Not only does this application fall within our definition of ideology, but, as applied to collectivities, it is increasingly political.[5]

This definition of invisible ideology fits well the history of gerontology in the last three decades. Social gerontology has always understood itself to be an application of science to social affairs in commitment to the rational improvement of the condition of the aged in modern society. Few people have questioned or challenged the desirability of that commitment. After all, who could be against helping the elderly? But the values presupposed by such an engagement of science on behalf of helping the elderly have rarely been held up to scrutiny. Science, like benevolent social action, is also likely to include elements of self-interest and ideology. The role of social science and the shape of public benevolence toward the aging also encompass elements of self-interest and ideology. But the relationships between science and values, between interest and ideology, have rarely been made explicit in aging policy.

One purpose or function of ideology is to contain contradictions that threaten to overwhelm social stability. These contradictions are reflected in the structure of ideological thought itself. At times, ideological constructions of social reality will present a pessimistic image of things: for example, the popularity of the Malthusian doctrine on population or the rise of Social Darwinism in the later 19th century. These pessimistic images had the effect of reinforcing the power of existing institutions or legitimating new forms of control. Pessimism implied that efforts to change the situation were hopeless. At the same time, there can be optimistic or positive constructions of social reality: for example, the concept of progress through technology or the idea of guaranteed legal rights. Such positive images of society also perform an ideological function by persuading people that all is well or is becoming better. What is important to emphasize here is the central role of contradiction or dialectic in social change and the role of ideology in legitimating existing institutions.

The framework of ideology in social change can be applied directly to the condition of old age and aging policy in America today. First, there are profound economic and technological forces at work: the changing nature of the labor market as we move toward an information economy and a post-industrial society; the impact of medical technology in prompting a demographic explosion of the "old-old"; the inadequate and inequitable financing of public and private pension systems at a time of growing life expectancy. As in the industrial revolution, new technological and economic forces bring about changes in the relations of production. The most visible of these has been the institution of retirement and the persistent problems of unemployment in advanced industrial society.

The effect of these economic and technological changes is that the elderly have become a "surplus population" without any role in the productivity of society. But these developments have affected different groups of the elderly in very different ways. Some groups have benefited, others have been harmed. Steven Crystal has characterized these as the "two worlds of aging": one well-to-do, healthy and in a favorable position, the other, poor, chronically ill, and suffering from many social problems of old age.[6] The increased size of *both* groups in recent years has been extraordinary. But our ideological construction of old age remains caught in a contradiction. One image of old age portrays the elderly as dependent and deserving of social services, but the design of those services may even increase their dependency. Another image of old age portrays the elderly as healthier, living longer, and leading active, happy lives. There are groups of old people who match either set of descriptions, but the two descriptions together are evidently in opposition. Like 19th century industrial society, we have a contradictory image of the social change we are undergoing. Both pessimism and optimism can have an ideological function of supporting the status quo and suppressing recognition of the dialectical structure—the inherent contradictions—of the ideology of old age.[7] The result is to suppress not only deeper knowledge but to overlook new sources of productivity and vitality in an aging population.

Motives for Ideology. Clifford Geertz has emphasized the complex character of ideological systems, above all, their ability to incorporate contradictory elements. Geertz observes that there are two main approaches to ideology: the interest theory and the strain theory. For interest theory, "ideology is a mask and a weapon," for the strain theory "a symptom and a remedy." He continues: "In the interest theory, ideological pronouncements are seen against the background of a universal struggle for advantage; in the strain theory, against the background of a chronic effort to correct sociopsychological disequilibrium."[8] The interest theory of ideology goes back to Marx and the class struggle; the strain theory goes back to Freud, to the process of denial and wish-fulfillment: "Ideology bridges the emotional gap between things as they are and as one would have them be. . ."[9] The interest theory explains the role of ideology in political tactics; the strain theory points to self-delusion and the dynamics of group solidarity in political movements.

In the politics of old age, we can expect to find ideology serving both functions of this kind. Some ideological discourse acts as a weapon for gaining advantage in political struggle and trade-off. For example, how the consumer price index measures the effect of inflation or poverty among the elderly is not merely an academic exercise. It can immediately become a weapon in the political arena. But other expressions of ideological thinking—such as the struggle of aging advocates against mandatory retirement—are best understood, not as tactics in a war of ideas, but as expressions of deep longings and symbolic aspirations. Such ideological expressions embody the contradictory images of old age in contemporary society. The struggle among competing ideologies of old age expresses the contradiction in still different forms.

The importance of the ideology of old age in political struggle today should not be underestimated. In the current political environment we have, since 1980, witnessed the triumph of a very clear-cut ideology in the Presidency of Ronald Reagan. That ideology appeals to deep American values such as self-reliance, personal responsibility, autonomy, and, above all, a desire for optimism and cheerful hope in the future. This constellation of values has been a key element in the public image and the appeal of Ronald Reagan. Liberals, including advocates for the aged, have tended to disregard the values of personal responsibility and optimism. But the strength of the Reagan program was based on much more than a public-relations appeal. It was based as well on the rise, during the 1970's, of well-financed conservative "think tanks," such as the American Enterprise Institute, the Hoover Institution, and the Heritage Foundation. These intellectual groups took very seriously the demanding task of fashioning a conservative mode of policy analysis. They succeeded in creating an intellectual alternative to the liberal consensus.

Until the 1980 election and the Reagan Administration, many liberals disregarded the question of ideology altogether, believing, perhaps complacently, that a "policy-based incrementalism" would sustain bipartisan commitment to the welfare state into the indefinite future. This failure to take ideology seriously, I would argue, was a crucial strategic error. By the 1984 election, liberals were scrambling to come up with a viable program of positive alternatives to the well-designed Reagan program. In the politics and ideology of old age, the same disregard for ideology and ideological criticism has been evident among liberal advocates for the elderly. To understand that failure, we need to look briefly at the rise of old age interest groups and the evolution of their ideology in the political arena.

THE AGING INTEREST GROUPS

In examining the ideology of old age we need to identify those periods of recent history when aging interest groups reached a measure of influence: that is, when ideology and organizational politics worked as powerful currents to advance the welfare of the elderly population. I refer here to the emergence of what Pratt has called a "Gray Lobby"—that collection of Washington-based aging interest groups whose activities have been documented by a number of political scientists.[10] The power and proliferation of current aging interest groups dates largely from the sixties, a decade that saw the widest influence of liberal ideology. The leadership of organizations in the Gray Lobby followed a strategy that paralleled other successful interest groups: calling attention to injustice and unmet needs, mobilizing political involvement by constituents, building alliances with other interest groups.

From an historical point of view, the emergence of a potent gray lobby in the seventies was somewhat anomalous.[11] The only previous time when old age politics had actually reached the scale of mass political mobilization occurred during the Depression years of the thirties. Significantly, it was during the thirties that old age politics incorporated a strongly expressed ideology of old age as seen in a number of powerful social movements on behalf of the elderly. Indeed, historians have noted that the original Social Security legislation, a centerpiece of the New Deal, was drafted in such a way as to take the steam out of the growing Townsend Movement. After 1940, the Townsend Movement progressively declined. Throughout the forties and fifties, old age politics lacked either a mass or an effective organizational base. Ideology was largely dormant, although the policy framework, principally Social Security, remained intact and continued its incremental expansion.[12]

In the 1960's the picture changed again. By the early fifties the National Council on Aging had been established and the American Association of Retired Persons began its process of growth. By the mid-sixties, the ideological climate had changed and claims of social justice could be advanced on behalf of the aged. Groups like NCOA and AARP took up the cause. Meanwhile, for the first time since the thirties, major federal policy initiatives in aging took place. Nineteen sixty-five, a high water mark of the Great Society, saw the landmark passage of Medicare and the establishment of the Administration on Aging. Medicare was important because it established a fundamental principle of government support for vital services to the elderly, while the Administration on Aging, and its allied network of state and local agencies, took up the mission of advocacy within the structure of government itself. While aging interest groups could not claim exclusive credit for these achievements, the Gray Lobby was vocal and visible and would from now on be in a position to advance ideological claims about the situation of old age in American society. But the ideology of old age articulated by the interest groups was different in style and sophistication from the global ideological aspirations of old age movements of the thirties. The ideological claims supported by aging interest groups in the sixties and seventies were closely integrated with the organizational structure of aging interest groups and their goals.

The organizational base for such claims was becoming more secure through the growth of interest groups themselves. NCOA began to grow in size and sophistication as it was supported by a variety of substantial federal grants and contracts. AARP, on the other hand, achieved its growth through services—such as publications and insurance—available to its membership, which exploded in size until AARP reached over ten million members by the 1980's. Other Gray Lobby organizations drew their strength from traditional alliances with other interest groups: the National Council of Senior Citizens had strong ties with the labor movement, Green Thumb with agricultural interests. All these groups flourished from government grants and contracts. By the time of the 1981 White House Conference with Aging, there were twenty six major aging interest groups which banded together to constitute a "Leadership Council of Aging Organizations." At the White House Conference the Leadership Council commanded public press attention, while behind the scenes maneuvered to rebuff the Reagan Administration's efforts to take control of events at the Conference.

In the "golden age" of aging policy—roughly 1965 to 1981— there was little need to be explicit about ideology. The elderly were a favored social welfare constituency; no politicians proposed to take away benefits from this group. The only question was what benefits would be added. It was in that period of rising entitlements that the prevailing ideological view of aging politics took shape. It was during this period that a consensus, a "social construction of reality" about old age, was arrived at. Of course, there is no single construction of an image of old age but rather an ongoing ideological contention about the "facts" of old age: Is aging a disease? Are old people poorer than other groups? Why do some elderly, but not others, take advantage of service programs that are available? The "facts" about old age are rarely clear. Ideological contention about those facts is what inspires a large body of research in social gerontology. That contention deeply affects not only politics or service delivery but even the scientific study of aging itself. In this competition among rival ideological constructions of social reality, there are many actors. The media, the academic community, political interest groups, and advocates for special causes all have had a share in defining the terms of the debate. This is true in the field of aging as it is for every other area of domestic policy. And, here too, ideology has the inevitable effect of suppressing facts that are inconsistent with the image of the problem set before us.

IDEOLOGY AND THE POLITICS OF AGING TODAY

How would we characterize the competing ideologies of old age today? For the last decade, the dominant ideological view of aging in America has been the liberal ideology. The liberal ideological view of aging sees old age as a social problem. The liberal mood of social crisis is captured well by the title and the message of Robert Butler's Pulitzer Prize winning book, *Why Survive?* The book documents a long litany of problems suffered by the elderly in America. Old people are subject to crime, inflation, poor health care, decay of the family—problems which in fact are widespread in our society but are thought intolerable for the elderly.

The liberal ideological view of aging has been picked up as a dominant theme by the mass media, by academic gerontology, by aging interest groups, and by the public at large, and survey research seems to confirm that public opinion sees older people with more "problems" than older people see themselves.[13] The liberal ideological view of aging has had an important effect on policy-making and on legislation. The early battles of that liberal ideological struggle were fought during the 1960's. In the mid-sixties, when the official "War on Poverty" became institutionally embodied in the old Office of Economic Opportunity, aging advocates proposed that the elderly too should have their special agency.

The Older Americans Act (1965) created the Administration on Aging and, over time, authorized a series of additional programs: Meals-on-Wheels, neighborhood Senior Citizens Centers, information and referral agencies, and a network of Area Agencies on Aging that operate through state and local government across the United States. While never commanding vast resources, this aging network did insure that a cadre of advocates and allies of aging interest groups would remain in place to press for the concerns of older Americans.[14] In that sense, the liberal ideological view of old age acquired a permanent niche within the federal system and the policy process. Most of the executive agencies and special programs of the Great Society legislation have disappeared but aging programs have remained. Compared to other social welfare programs, services for the aging have flourished. Every few years the reauthorization of the Older Americans Act offers an opportunity for the symbolic politics that is an important element of the liberal ideological view.[15]

The script for this ritual is by now familiar. The old are cast in the role of the deserving poor. The problems of old age are recited and duly noted by organs of official opinion. Nursing home scandals or crime against the elderly make the headlines. Editorials are written; legislative hearings are scheduled; public officials are interviewed. Before long, there is general public consensus that "something must be done." Protective legislation and health or welfare appropriations follow in due course. In broad terms, this is the familiar rhythm of the liberal policy process. In good times, it is the basis for policy-based incrementalism to add new benefits and entitlements; in bad times, the "plight of the aged" becomes a rallying point for resisting budget cuts.

The "Failure Model" of Old Age. But a certain undercurrent in the liberal policy process must be noted. The process is a success only to the extent that the condition of old age is presented as a failure. The liberal ideological policy stance is directly linked with what Kalish has called the "failure model" of aging.[16] The failure model sees old age as a period of decline and disaster. The ideological power of the liberal ideology necessarily casts old people as the deserving poor, as helpless, even pathetic victims requiring our protection: "Grandma Found Beaten and Robbed," "Old Folks Forced to Steal from Supermarkets," "Aged Eating Dogfood," "Goldenview Nursing Home Cited for Filthy Conditions." These are familiar phrases from the headlines, guaranteed to provoke moral outrage. It is this image that sells newspapers, that wins elections, that supports enlarged budgets for police departments, social service staff, and gerontological professionals whose livelihood depends on the credibility of this ideology.

Even "enlightened" opinion holds fast to the belief that the elderly, unlike others, are forced to live on "fixed incomes" or that old people are in trouble because of a decline in the "extended family." Pseudoscientific jargon like "fixed income" or "extended family" is repeated mindlessly. The jargon betrays the way in which conventional wisdom on old age is the residue of falsifications and distortions that support an ideological construction of the position of old people. In the face of this negative image, it is not surprising that only the very poor come forward to identify themselves as "old" when polled on the subject.[17] After all, it is more respectable to be "retired" than to be labelled "unemployed." Only for the poor does identification with old age mean any sort of positive status. The success of this ideological construction of the image of old age is the spread of a certain "false consciousness" even among the bulk of the elderly themselves: if I am old and doing relatively well, then I judge myself an "exception" to the general state of disaster that old age in America is held to be.[18]

CHALLENGE TO THE LIBERAL DEFINITION OF THE "AGING PROBLEM"

Who are the principal beneficiaries of the liberal ideological view of aging? Certainly old people themselves benefit from such things as indexing of Social Security payments. But the providers of services to the elderly also benefit; for example, hospitals and health professionals benefit from Medicare. Emphasizing the decremental or failure model of aging provides justification for public subsidies that might otherwise be cut. Some may know it's an exaggeration, but it is difficult to admit that in public. Indeed, the liberal ideological definition of the "aging problem" is widely shared by all elements of the major old age organizations existing in Washington: i.e., those groups banded together under the Leadership Council of Aging Organizations. The point is not that such groups themselves have become part of an "Aging Enterprise" which benefits from government funding for services.[19] Direct patronage is only a modest element of the picture. Rather, in order to maintain their own internal legitimacy and to carry out their advocacy role representing their constituency, these aging advocacy groups are compelled to adopt a liberal "party line" on aging issues.[20]

Knowledgeable people recognize, of course, many facts inconsistent with the liberal ideological view. Crime statistics suggest that the old are *less* likely than the young to be crime victims. Not all nursing homes are the chamber of horrors the public tends to believe. But in any case only 5% of the elderly reside in nursing homes, whatever their quality. And as a result of indexing Social Security against inflation, the proportion of the old who are below the poverty line has dropped dramatically over the last two decades. At least until quite recently, the old were less likely than the young to be below the poverty level.[21] These facts may not be appreciated by public opinion. The facts may be passed over by the prevailing liberal ideology but the facts are now becoming well known to policy-makers and policy influentials.

Neoconservative View of Old Age. What about the neoconservative view of aging? It is a striking fact that until quite recently, it was difficult to find strongly expressed conservative views about old age policy. There was a time, during the thirties, when aging policy, in particular pensions and social security, were matters of intense ideological debate. Oddly enough, it was in the United States, not in other countries, where such topics became matters of ideological controversy.[22] But in recent years the ideological debate receded and the vacuum of conservative ideology on old age policy is striking. The situation is all the more strange since on all other matters of domestic policy, clear-cut ideological differences abound. On crime, for instance, or education, or race relations, there has long been an articulate neoconservative viewpoint represented, for example, in the pages of *The Public Interest* or *Commentary* magazines. New policy proposals on the family or welfare reform or urban policy were sure to receive critical examination from both a liberal and a conservative point of view. Not so for aging policy. To the extent that consensus liberal politics held sway, the liberal view has dominated public opinion on the issue.

This strange silence and monolithic ideological agreement has not necessarily been beneficial. In a way it is all too reminiscent of the late fifties when Daniel Bell wrote his famous book *The End of Ideology* and declared the end of fundamental political debate in the United States. According to Bell and his colleague Seymour Martin Lipset "the fundamental political problems. . . have been solved." In place of the old ideological and intellectual rivalries of the thirties and forties—generally linked to the Old Left—a new, modernized America had transcended ideology in favor of a pragmatic style of technical rationality in the solution of social problems. As Michael Rogin notes, the Bell-Lipset version of the end of ideology "in fact justified the instrumentalist thinking by which a new, bureaucratic middle class served the dominant structures of power in American life."[23] The so-called end of ideology was a disguise and an evasion. Widespread silence was an ominous absence of critical thought concerning central matters of public policy. Something of the same development has occurred during the "golden age" of aging policies from the mid-sixties until the early 1980's. During that period, a consensus liberal politics of aging also held sway. In the growth of "aging network" as well as in incrementalist Social Security policy, the style of technical rationality and pragmatic problem-solving carried the day.

Liberal ideology easily "captured" debate on old age policy because most political actors held an essentially benevolent and generous view of the elderly as a social welfare constituency. In addition, conservative spokesmen often appeared outmoded, unintelligent, and hidebound. But with the rise of an intellectually articulate neoconservative ideology in recent years, major elements of the entire liberal consensus have come under attack. For example, on criminal justice policy, it is no longer "obvious" to informed opinion that rehabilitation is to be favored over punishment. And, in aging policy too, there are now voices that have been raised to criticize the liberal consensus that earlier held sway.

The lines of a neoconservative view on old age policy have been proposed by Rabushka and Jacobs in *Old Folks at Home.*[24] The authors focus heavily on housing policy for the elderly, where they note that 80% of older people own their own homes and thus are shielded from the high mortgage rates of recent years. But Rabushka and Jacobs develop a more extended neoconservative argument against familiar liberal complaints about the dismal condition of older Americans. In sum, Rabushka and Jacobs claim the complaints are vastly exaggerated and frequently just plain wrong. Basically, the neoconservative view argues that, when multiple transfer payments and subsidies are taken into account, old people today, in economic terms, really aren't badly off. Compared to other groups in the population, in fact, the elderly are doing reasonably well.

Support for the neoconservative position comes from the 1982 data of the U.S. Census. The figures indicate the dramatic and continuing drop in the poverty rate among the elderly since the mid-sixties. At that time the poverty among older people was twice that of the general population. By 1982, the poverty rate among the old was no greater than any other group and in fact perhaps lower if in-kind (noncash) benefits are taken into account. In recent years, the elderly coped well with economic distress, as the Census Bureau suggests. Since most people over 65 are retired, high unemployment rates didn't affect them, while Social Security benefits and some other benefits are indexed to shield them from inflation. The most ominous element of the new poverty statistics is the dramatic surge in the poverty rate for children. Critics who are unhappy with the age-based entitlements for the elderly can point to these statistics for additional support for their position that the old are no worse off than other groups.

Recent Eclipse of the Liberal View of Old Age. If the neoconservative view is correct, then it's hard to see why the elderly, as a group, should be entitled to special benefit programs under public policy. The neoconservative analysis is a rationale for cutting age-based entitlements and replacing them with programs based on need, perhaps employing a means test to target services to the truly needy. Some such view has often been heard from the Reagan Administration. But the same view is echoed by some gerontologists, such as Bernice Neugarten in her call for an "age-irrelevant" society where age-based entitlements to special services will be replaced by services provided according to need, not chronological age.[25] While the age-need debate has often been conducted among academic gerontologists, the Social Security funding crisis brought wider calls to cut back entitlements for the elderly. Critics argued that the Social Security system itself is unfairly subsidizing older people at the expense of other groups in the population and other pressing economic needs.

This ideological stance suggests that benefit and subsidy programs for the old can be cut or perhaps converted entirely to means-tested programs.[26] The gains of efficiency by cutting overall cost would be matched by gains in fundamental equity allowing us to help the truly needy first. Meeting the twin goals of efficiency and equity has great appeal and probably helped the Reagan Administration in its struggle to end the Social Security minimum benefit. How could liberals be against the policy of targeting welfare resources at the most needy groups? That policy debate underscored the ideological significance of past aging policies that were grounded in a view of the aging as the deserving poor. The empirical question became the issue of how far the elderly poor would be hurt, whether they could be aided under SSI, and so on. Obviously, the neoconservative ideology will emphasize an image of old people as relatively well off and therefore unlikely to be harmed by cuts in public entitlement programs.

The shift away from the liberal ideological view of the aging found its clearest expression in the bipartisan "compromise" on Social Security, engineered in January, 1983. For the first time, leaders of both parties acknowledged the need to cut benefit increases in the future. Moreover, provisions for taxing Social Security benefits were a form of "backdoor" general revenue support for the System. General revenue support for Social Security had long been on the liberal agenda and was now to be accompanied by additional benefit provisions for SSI. Some aging advocacy groups, such as AARP, opposed the taxation of any social security benefits for older people, even for those with high income. But the final legislation amounted to an acknowledgement that, in fact, the elderly are not all needy and deserving of public subsidy. By taxing the benefits of the more well-to-do elderly, the Social Security program in effect introduced a needs-based criterion as against age-based entitlements which had been the core of the program. At the same time, the Social Security compromise agreement did little to curb the rising pressure on the Medicare Trust Fund and so the need for cost containment in health care will continue to be an issue in the future.[27] Despite the fading of the Social Security "crisis," the ideological struggle over aging policy is bound to continue in the future.

Ideological Struggle: The Uncertain Future. A well-defined liberal and conservative ideology of old age has emerged sharply only in very recent years. It remains to be seen how the ideological realignment will play itself out, but some directions are clear. Any national administration will face pressures for cost containment in health care and social services for the aging in the foreseeable future. At the same time, the prospect of recovery from the recession is likely to mean a high level of unemployment for years to come. The highest rates of unemployment will be concentrated, disproportionately, among older workers and minority youth. The "broad brush" ideological view of old-time liberalism, the view of the aged as the deserving poor, may become untenable, even by liberals.[28] In this sense, the neoconservatives have won. They have put liberalism on the defensive by redefining the terms of the debate. The question of "Who are the deserving poor?" will surface again and again and make allocation based on need a challenge for the future.

The ideological struggle endures but now the struggle is pursued in a more covert way. In the new environment, the "graying of the Federal budget" means that policymakers must increasingly pursue the goals of cost containment and service reduction in a fashion that is covert and indirect.[29] This was the lesson learned by the Reagan Administration after its first bumbling, and disastrous, attempt to reform Social Security in 1981. Social Security thereafter became a hot potato to be handled only by a covert ideological struggle waged behind closed doors of a bipartisan National Commission. The technique of appointing a blue-ribbon Commission, as in the case of the MX missile or the Kissinger Commission on Central America, was no mere exercise in symbolic politics. It was a successful attempt to insulate real policy-making from public opinion and the Congress, where "policy paralysis" seemed unavoidable.

The Reagan Administration's successful displacement of ideological struggle to an offstage Commission set the pattern for further behind-the-scenes policy development. Further changes in policy on Medicare and Medicaid would also come about through covert means: by regulatory change and quiet rule-making or by covert administrative acts invisible from public scrutiny. Political leaders feel they cannot afford to offend the aged constituency by pursuing goals of cost-containment overtly. Still less can they move explicitly toward needs-tested and means-tested programs for the elderly. But behind the scenes a historical shift between overt and covert policy-making in aging policy is now occurring.

This balance between an overt and covert ideology of old age has a long history. Indeed, outright controversy which entails "politicizing" old age to the point where an actual "old age movement" might is extremely rare. The most prominent, some would say unique, example in American history occurred during the 1930's with the Townsend Movement and similar phenomena. But a *covert* ideological development has been underway for some time. It is this covert ideological development and its history that must be understood. Cole observes that "By the mid-20th century, the outlines of a professional aging industry began to take shape in major urban areas across the country."[30] Like any industry, this "Aging Enterprise" (Estes) developed an ideology that serves as a rational justification for interest group concerns. Indeed, Cole's historical analysis corrects and enlarges Estes' account by locating the system of aging services in institutions whose power long preceded the Older Americans Act: institutions like the hospital, the life insurance industry, or the funeral industry. A spectrum of interest groups has served the needs of the elderly and an ideological structure supported those groups.

But unlike most other interest groups, the needs of the aging have been relatively uncontroversial. Compared to minorities, the unemployed, families with dependent children, or other needy groups, the elderly have been a favored and uncontroversial constituency. The old were regarded as "deserving": no one could be blamed for growing old. Thus, the ideological controversy over helping the aged was muted. Partly for this reason, the ideology of old age has been invisible, rarely debated. Quietly, without public fanfare, the aging industry has advanced its organizational claims over new questions of how the needs of later life would be met. The life insurance industry, hospitals and nursing homes, professionals in health care and social welfare have all seen their power grow proportionately. Allied sectors, such as travel, retirement housing, or the leisure-time industry have benefited too. In this historical development, government, the professions, and academia each played a role. But in constructing and legitimating professional intervention, ideological contradictions were suppressed. In recent history, those contradictions have emerged again as a more powerful and articulate "Gray Lobby" played its role in Washington.

Origins of the Gray Lobby. The so-called "Gray Lobby"—interest group organizations advocating on behalf of the elderly had grown up during the 1920's and reached the proportions of a social movement during the Depression. But the flowering of "interest group liberalism" tied to old age came only in the 1960's and after. The pattern of successful advocacy was shown by other disadvantaged groups, above all by the civil rights movement of the sixties. Using the same broad strategy, aging interest groups cast the elderly in the image of a minority group or a status of intrinsic disadvantage. This strategy and rhetoric worked, as Achenbaum noted:

> The elderly 'fit' into the Great Society mold. The 'problem' of old age was perceived as a legitimate 'welfare' issue. The aged's needs could be reduced by increasing categorical allocations and inaugurating new social services. By presenting their case in politically astute terms, the elderly were able to capitalize on the politics of interest group liberalism. They became entitled to more and more. The cost of aging programs rapidly became a major item in annual federal budgets.[31]

While conservative conventional wisdom is fond of insisting that the Great Society programs allegedly "failed," that view doesn't hold for old age programs at all. As the poverty statistics on the aging suggest, we are confronted by an embarrassing degree of success. The critical role was played by the ideology and programs of the Great Society legislation. Achenbaum, reviewing the recent history of federal policies in aging, takes note of the "central paradox" of Great Society legislation and its impact on aged: namely, that war-on-poverty programs eventually had greater benefit for the elderly than for the disadvantaged groups they were intended to address. This was not the purpose of the Great Society reformers at all.[32] Certainly the poverty of the elderly was highlighted, for example, in Harrington's *The Other America*. But the anti-poverty programs of the Johnson administration were primarily targeted at youth, minorities, the unemployed, and the rural and urban poor. Indeed, one of the motivations for the establishment of the Administration on Aging in 1965 was to create a parallel agency for the problems of the elderly, since it was assumed that the Office of Economic Opportunity, the flagship agency for anti-poverty efforts, would be likely to overlook the elderly in its focus on youth.

But the conclusion of this tale conveys its irony. While programs to aid the poor were attacked by Nixon, programs for the aged continued to grow and were not attacked. The ideology behind anti-poverty efforts was challenged from many quarters and suffered a decline throughout the seventies. By contrast, the ideology of old age, particularly the negative covert ideology, grew stronger all the time. Finally, twenty years later OEO and other federal anti-poverty initiatives had been swept away, while AoA's budget approached a billion dollars a year. The Reagan Administration succeeded in slashing benefit programs, especially means-tested programs, for the poor. But middle-class entitlement programs for the aged (Social Security, Medicare) were barely touched. The "two worlds" of aging moved ever farther apart. But in the prevailing ideology of old age, the elderly still retained their favored status. Even as shrewd an observer as Peter Clecak seems to believe that the Reagan program initiated significant cuts in government aid for "students, poor people, children, and old people."[33] The liberal litany here has a familiar ring. In fact Reagan did severely slash benefits for the first three groups, but *not* for the elderly—at least not until the Social Security compromise plan, which can hardly be laid entirely at the doorstep of Mr. Reagan. The belief that old people—the "deserving poor"— have been disproportionately harmed by Reagan's program dies hard.

Prospects for the Future. We need to recognize that under the Reagan budget cutbacks and economic policies, the elderly generally did far better than any other vulnerable group.[34] Yet despite their relative success, the political atmosphere had changed. The impact of the change in mood and prospects of the future will be felt for the remainder of the decade by aging interest groups. Unlike the 1970's, the 1980's will witness hard choices for aging interests. During the 1970's the position of the elderly improved markedly relative to other groups, and, during the first years of the Reagan counterrevolution, the elderly held their own. These successes could be claimed as victories by aging interest groups. But could these groups equally claim responsibility for the alternative of going along with cutbacks in entitlement programs? This alternative will be unpalatable, but now that the aging interest groups have become participants in the political bargaining process, it may prove harder to distance themselves from the outcome. The other alternative—to keep distance by maintaining the unbending rigor of advocacy—may mean that the key decisions (e.g., where to cut Medicare) are made without direct influence by the Gray Lobby at all.

What will be the role of aging interest groups in the future as they seek to influence the policy domain in health care, income, and other aging policy issues? During the seventies, aging interest groups could stake out different ideological positions: for example, AARP occupying a moderate position, while NCSC could articulate issues from a more traditional liberal-labor position. The coming of hard times has, on the one hand, brought the aging interests together, into the "common front" of the Leadership Council of Aging Organizations that was so active in the 1981 White House Conference on Aging. This common threat has demanded a subduing or blending of ideological differences. Yet, for all the reasons offered earlier, it may prove impossible to suppress indefinitely the contradictions embodied in the ideology of the aging interest groups. The most serious of these contradictions, of course, is economic or social class. The threat of divergent class interests was evident at the time of the compromise solution on Social Security financing—e.g., taxing Social Security benefits of higher income beneficiaries. These contradictions will reappear.

During the fifties and sixties other groups—such as organized labor, churches, and traditional social welfare constituencies—represented old people's interests. But momentum toward the "professionalization of reform" was already underway. By the end of the sixties, as aging interest groups expanded their numbers, size and visibility, the ideological agenda of these interest groups became defined and dominated by professionals. This was true even in a case where, like AARP, these groups had a large mass membership with active local chapters. With 14 million members by 1983, AARP alone could claim great political legitimacy when lobbying among legislators, quite apart from whether or not AARP, or any of the aging interest groups, could actually wield electoral power. But now we may witness the prospect of disenchantment by politicians with aging organizations on practical, not ideological grounds. The political question may be: can they really deliver the vote?[35] If the answer is no, then the real source of power among aging interests may come to depend more on agenda-setting than on bargaining from a presumed electoral power base. Here one should keep in mind the importance of an agenda-setting model in understanding the process of political change. By virtue of their history, visibility, and presumptive legitimacy, the aging interest groups will retain a degree of power to influence the definition of issues. Access to media, influence over public opinion, and possession of knowledge are critical assets here. But so too is ideological clarity and a sense of coherent goals and priorities. Here recent history does not provide grounds for optimism.

The Older Americans Act, including its major expansion with 1973 amendments, created what might be seen as an empty "policy space" for political action. But by the 1980's, this policy space had become filled up by a dense network of State and Area Agencies on Aging, each serving to coordinate other agencies and local interest groups. More seriously still, the emergent "aging network" entailed a subtle shift in the original intentions of the Older Americans Act. Originally given a mission of advocacy and agenda-setting, the aging network agencies have more and more become an alternate, age-based service delivery system. This transformation of role has meant a loss of ideological clarity among network agencies at lower levels of the system as well as the incorporation of local organizations (churches, neighborhood groups, voluntary agencies) that depend on government contracts to deliver services authorized under the Older Americans Act. "Mediating structures" have become integral elements of the service delivery pattern. In short, this alternate, age-based service system has become an interest-group in itself.

THE STRUCTURE OF THE IDEOLOGY OF OLD AGE

This historical background on the current politics of aging sets the stage for a more precise definition of the ideology of old age. The ideology of old age can be divided into two parts: a surface structure and a deep structure, or, as I shall call them here, the Overt Ideology and the Covert Ideology. The Overt Ideology is a system of ideas that are easily recognized and debated. The Overt Ideology of old age is constituted by the broad division between theory and practice, between knowledge and action. The contradictions of that ideology are bound up with a separation between those spheres of social life, and this separation generates contradictions familiar in other areas of social life. The Covert Ideology, on the other hand, is hidden, more involved in unconscious attitudes and stereotypes, with our hopes and fears. For example, the notion of "ageism," the psychology of age-identification, and ambiguous position of young people cast in the role of aging advocates or professional gerontologists; these are all instances involving deep contradictions that the Covert Ideology obscures and evades.

The overriding challenge of an aging society, I would argue, is not the struggle against ageism, not even the advocacy effort for social justice on behalf of the vulnerable elderly. Instead, the challenge is to a more fundamental struggle: to make conscious the contradictions and ideological deformations that paralyze action or distort communication.[36] The task is to bring together surface structure and deep structure, the overt and the covert ideology of old age. Only by moving toward consciousness and acknowledgement of contradiction can we hope for a society in which lifespan development is an ideal that can be embodied in major social institutions.

This task of reconstruction, I argue, cannot be accomplished on the model of the social sciences, including social gerontology, that now prevails. Instead, what is required is a "dialectical" gerontology. But to understand the need for the dialectic, we must understand the Overt and Covert ideology of old age today. The problem of understanding is made worse by the fact that many will deny that any ideology exists at all.

REFERENCES

1. For example, Ethel Shanas, "Social Myth as Hypothesis: The Case of the Family Relations of Old People," *Gerontologist*, 19:3-9 (1979).

2. Erdman Palmore, "Attitudes Toward the Aged," *Research on Aging*, 4:3 (1982), 333-48.

3. Clark Tibbitts, "Can We Invalidate Negative Stereotypes of Aging?" *The Gerontologist*, 4:3 (1979), 10-20.

4. Carroll Estes, J. Swan, and Gerard, "Dominant and Competing Paradigms in Gerontology: Towards a Political Economy of Ageing," *Ageing and Society*, 2:2 (1982), 285-98.

5. David Apter, *Ideology and Discontent*, New York, Free Press, 1964, p. 17. Apter admits that this way of putting the matter can be "troublesome" because it extends our ordinary notions of ideology into new areas." The current chapter is an effort to extend this concept of ideology into the field of aging.

6. Steven Crystal, *America's Old Age Crisis: Public Policy and the Two Worlds of Aging,* New York, Basic Books, 1982.

7. On ideology see Karl Marx, *The German Ideology* and *The Holy Family*; George Lichtheim, *Marxism: An Historical and Critical Study,* London, 1961. Seliger, Martin, *The Marxist Conception of Ideology: A Critical Essay.* London, 1977. In the American context, see Everett Carl Ladd, *Ideology in America.* Cornell Univ. Press, 1963; Morris Janowitz, *The Last Half Century,* Univ. of Chicago Press; Irving Louis Horowitz, *Ideology and Utopia in the United States: 1956-1976,* New York, Oxford University Press, 1977.

8. Clifford Geertz, "Ideology as a Cultural System," pp.47-76 in David Apter, *Ideology and Discontent,* New York, Free Press, 1964, p.52.

9. Ibid., p.55.

10. Henry J. Pratt, *The Grey Lobby,* 1976. More recently, Hudson, Robert B. (ed.), *The Aging in Politics: Process and Policy,* Springfield, Charles C. Thomas, 1981.

11. David H. Fischer, "The Politics of Aging: A Short History," *Jour. of the Institute for Socioeconomic Studies,* 4:2 (1979), 51-66.

12. Sara Alice Rosenberry, *The Role of Ideology in Policy Development: A Comparison of British and American Old Age Income Security Efforts,* Rutgers Univ. Press, 1980.

13. Louis Harris & Associates, *The Myth and Reality of Aging in America* (Washington, DC, National Council on Aging, 1977). The extraordinary gap between public perception and reality is discussed by Douglas McAdam, "Coping with Aging.or Combating Ageism?" in Aliza Kolker and Paul I. Ahmed, *Aging.* New York, Elsevier, 1982.

14. Donald Gelfand, *The Aging Network.*

15. Murray Edelman, *The Symbolic Uses of Politics,* Urbana, Univ. of Illinois Press, 1967.

16. Richard A. Kalish, "The New Ageism and the Failure Models: A Polemic," *The Gerontologist,* (1979), Vol. 19, pp. 175-202.

17. See analysis of Harris survey data by Menachem Daum, "Preferences for Age-Mixed Social Interaction," in B. Neugarten (ed.), *Age of Need? Public Policies for Older People,* Sage Publications, 1982.

18. H.J. O'Gorman, "False Consciousness of Kind: Pluralistic Ignorance among the Aged," *Research on Aging,* 2:1 (1980), 105-128.

19. Douglas McAdam, "Coping with Aging or Combating Ageism?" in Aliza Kolker and Paul I. Ahmed, *Aging.* New York, Elsevier, 1982. McAdam, echoing Estes (*The Aging Enterprise*) seems to intimate that large numbers of service personnel—including academic gerontologists—benefit from the "service strategy" linked to a liberal ideological view of old age. There is no question that such financial interests play a role in the budgets of aging advocacy organizations—of AARP or NCOA—just as government funding does for hospitals, physicians, insurance companies, and so on. But the history of the liberal ideological view of aging advocacy organizations long predates the availability of government funding. We don't really require such grossly material influences to explain the persistence of the ideology in any case. On the contrary, what demands explanation is the strength and persistence of such views among intellectuals, policy influentials and groups who derive no benefit from the funding of state-supported services.

20. Henry J. Pratt, "Politics of Aging: Political Science and the Study of Gerontology," *Research on Aging,* Vol. 1, No.2 (June, 1979).

21. For a discussion of the role of ideological elements in shaping the way "poverty" is defined and measured among the elderly, see Lori Gershick and John Williamson, "The Politics of Measuring Poverty among the Elderly," *Policy Studies Journal,* Vol. 10, No. 3 (Mar., 1982), 483-499.

22. Anthony King, "Ideas, Institutions and the Policies of Governments: A Comparative Analysis, Parts I and II, *British Jour. of Political Science,* 3 (1973), pp. 302-313. See also Anthony King, "The Political Consequences of the Welfare State," in Shimon Spiro and Ephraim Yuchtman-Yaar (eds.), *Evaluating the Welfare State: Social and Political Perspectives,* New York, Academic Press, 1983.

23. Michael Rogin, "In Defense of the New Left," *Democracy,* Vol. 3, No. 4, Fall 1983, pp.106-116.

24. Alvin Rabushka and Bruce Jacobs, *Old Folks at Home.* For another neoconservative analysis (though not primarily of aging programs), see Jack A. Meyer (ed.), *Meeting Human Needs: Toward a New Public Philosophy,* Washington, D.C., American Enterprise Institute, 1982.

25. Bernice L. Neugarten, *Age or Need? Public Policies for Older People,* Beverly Hills, Sage Publications, 1982. Prof. Neugarten herself is the most prominent gerontologist who has called for more consideration of moving from chronological age to need as a basis for allocating services. Strangely enough, Neugarten has developed her position without any self-conscious commitment to a conservative ideology on aging policy. Her purely "academic" conclusions turn out to have surprising congruence with renewed calls for means-testing aging programs. Her position shows how the lack of self-conscious critique of ideology in gerontology may turn into a strange alliance with the forces of the political Right, which of course was not Neugarten's purpose at all.

26. Elizabeth Kutza, *The Benefits of Old Age: Social-Welfare Policy for the Elderly,* Chicago, Univ. of Chicago Press, 1981. Kutza, like Neugarten, calls into question the historical liberal commitment to age-categorical entitlement programs. She suggests that more effective means-testing could allocate limited resources to those elderly in greatest need.

27. J.K. Inglehart, "The Cost of Keeping the Elderly Well," *National Journal,* 10 (1978), 1728-31.

28. Kutza, op. cit.

29. Robert B. Hudson, "The Graying of the Federal Budget and Its Consequences for Old Age Policy," *The Gerontologist,* 18(5) (Oct., 1978), 428-440.

30. Thomas Cole, "The Ideology of Old Age and Death in American History," *American Quarterly,* XXXI, 2 (Summer, 1979), 223-231.

31. W. Andrew Achenbaum, *Shades of Grey,* Boston, Little, Brown, 1982, p.116.

32. Ibid., p.128.

33. Peter Clecak, *America's Quest for the Ideal Self,* p.332.

34. James Storey, *Older Americans in the Reagan Era: Impacts of Federal Policy Changes,* Urban Institute Press, 1983.

35. What Robert Binstock calls the "electoral bluff." Cf. Binstock, Robert, "Interest-Group Liberalism and the Politics of Aging," *The Gerontologist,* 12, 1972, pp. 265-280.

36. This theme of "distorted communications" that prevent human fulfillment is the leit-motif of the critical theory of Jurgen Habermas. Cf. *Legitimation Crisis* (trans. Thomas McCarthy), Boston, Beacon Press, 1975. For commentary on Habermas, see Anthony Giddens, *Central Problems in Social Theory,* Univ. of Calif. Press, 1979; J. Thompson, and D. Held, *Habermas: Critical Debates*; Thomas McCarthy, *The Critical Theory of Jurgen Habermas,* MIT Press, 1978.

Section II

UNDERSTANDING THE DOMAIN
OF GERONTOLOGICAL
COMMUNITY PRACTICE

Chapter III

Understanding Normative Growth and Development in Aging: Working With Strengths

Margaret E. Hartford

Every day about 5000 people reach the age of 65 in the United States, while 3,400 people over the age of 65 die. Obviously the older population continues to increase in size each year. While statistics quickly become obsolete, it is noteworthy that the 1980 census data showed 11.5% of the population, or over 25 million people were in the senior age bracket. These people range from 65 to 110; the youngest age grouping of old age ranging from 65 to 74 is the largest proportion of this population 62%; the middle old 75-84 28%, and the old old 85 to 95 8.4%, and now an increasing population of very old 95-105 the centenarians.

Each new generation is reaching old age in better health, with more education, higher economic status, and with considerable energy to continue to contribute to the well being of society, their communities, their families, and the maintenance of themselves. What they lack, if anything, is the opportunity to continue to be involved in the mainstream of American life. but this too is changing as the network of linkages among older adults becomes stronger, and they begin to create their own systems of participation, and as they take more responsibility for advocacy to create and protect their own rights.

Most of the people over 65 are physically well and mentally competent and able to function independently. While a high proportion of older adults have one or more chronic diseases, arthritis, heart disease, respiratory ailments, digestive problems, 80% of the people over 65 are not substantially restricted by illnesses.

The majority of adults 65 and older in the United States are in the category of the "well elderly." Between 80 and 90% of older people are well functioning, moderately healthy or coping with their chronic illnesses, socially competent and managing their own lives. Ninety percent of these people live independently in their own homes, or in homes with relatives or friends (U.S. Census Bureau, 1978). The other 10% of the well elderly live in various types of retirement communities, or in rental property where they can maintain independent living. Only 10 to 20% of older adults are defined as frail and dependent, cared for in hospitals, nursing homes, partial or total care facilities or are living with relatives where they require special care. Of the elderly only approximately 5% is institutionalized at any one time.

In a recent survey of the noninstitutionalized older people, 69% reported that their health was good or excellent, 22% reported that their health was fair and 9% reported that it was poor. If the 9% who reported poor health is added to the 5% who are institutionalized because of poor physical or mental health about 14% of older people are in poor health. While 80% of the people living in the community reported some chronic health problem, less than 18% said it limited their mobility (Brotman, 1980).[1]

Older adults in the United States reflect a diverse population by age cohort, sex, race, cultural heritage, socioeconomic level, personality characteristics, intellectual capacity and life style. They reflect all of the characteristics of the total population, except that they have survived to an old age and consequently have experienced a social history of the dramatic technological and social changes in the past 60 to 100 years.

In this chapter we will consider some of the characteristics of the older population, and the individual differences within it, some of the aspects of the normal aging process for people in their 60s, 70s, 80s, and 90s, some of the factors effecting longevity and life expectancy, some of the stresses of growing older in our society, some of the needs of older adults which may be met through the various types of social welfare services. By social services we refer to those programs focusing on prevention, support, engagement and involvement, rehabilitation and maintenance of individuals and families, and also program design, development, planning and organization of the aging services network.

AGE COHORT CHARACTERISTICS

Recognizing that people born within a decade of each other have shared some of the same experiences, and also seem to have similar characteristics, social psychologists came up with the concept of "aging cohorts." Neugarten[2] (1972) developed the classification of the young old 65 to 74 years of age, the middle old 75 to 84, and the old old 85 to 90s. Today one might add a fourth cohort, the very old, the centenarians of which estimates range from 30,000 to 100,000 in the U.S. Cain (1980)[3] also developed some of the characteristics of each cohort based on social and cultural events that conditioned their experiences.

The Young Old

The majority (62%) of older adults fall within the young old cohort group. They are newly retired people or those still employed full or part-time. Where persons have continued to work, they are the senior workers in business, professions, industry, labor, the arts, and in organizations, unions and government. While in some instances they have moved into senior leadership roles, offering consultation, wisdom, creativity and initiative, in other instances they have moved to lesser responsibility and lesser influence. With the extension of mandatory retirement from age 65 to age 70 in many categories of work, it is anticipated that more of the young old category will remain employed. The trend in the 1970's and early 1980's, however, in many categories of work, was for people of this cohort to take an early retirement, or to move to part time or split time employment. In business and industry where employment of older workers has been extended, or where retirees in this age category have been hired back, they have been found to be careful, competent, less prone to accidents and absenteeism than younger workers, and have demonstrated commitment and loyalty to their employers (McConnell, 1978),[4] as well as lending the perspective of their experience and wisdom.

The phenomenon of women outliving men begins to show in the young old cohort. In the age bracket 65 to 75 women have outlived men 130:100 (Brotman, 1980).[5]

The young old tend to be American born, though for a substantial number, their parents may have immigrated to the United States from many parts of the world in the 1890's to the 1920's. Within this cohort also are many people of foreign birth who comprised the waves of refugees who entered the United States in the '40's, during and after World War II.

An increasing proportion of the older population has had education in high school and college, though no statistics are available for specific cohorts over 65. In 1979 about 44% of the people over 65 had had less than a 10th grade education, but 9% were college graduates (Brotman, 1980),[6] and 23% had completed high school. Each succeeding generation has had more opportunity to attend school than their predecessors. The young old are the first generation to have benefited by the accessibility of low cost higher education through public education resources, the city and state financed college and university systems, the G.I. Bill after World War II benefitting servicemen, and extensive scholarship and loan funds.

Most of the young old continue to be active in their communities, in their organizations, with their families and friends, and some have continued to work full or part-time. Many have taken on volunteer roles, and others have increased their citizen participation, while others have increased their recreation and adult education activities. Perhaps one of the particular ways that social workers can assist people in this cohort is to help them to find new and inventive ways to develop functional roles in which to use their energy, talents, skills and abilities which are no longer utilized in the workplace, when they retire, or in families to the same extent as when their children were growing, or in organizations where younger leadership is competing to achieve and direct. Education, citizen roles and political activity, and community service appear to be the ways in which the young old cohort has thus far been connected with the wider society as they have left the employed work force.

One of the major categories of crises facing the young old and impacting this population greater than some of the other generations of older adults is the first recognition of compounded losses. Most people of the 65-75 age bracket are experiencing some functional loss through retirement of the occupations by which they defined themselves. With retirement also there is usually decrease in income estimated to be approximately one half to two thirds of earned income while employed. The loss of income may also mean a curtailment of certain social and recreational activities that were work or income related. Lodges, unions, service clubs or social clubs may be associated with jobs, and also affordable only with full income. Family patterns and relationships also frequently change during this decade of life as children move to their independent homes and families, and grandparent roles are not well defined in most American cultural populations. Death rates also increase rapidly for this age bracket, and the young old may notice for the first time the number of their peers, and especially men, who die within the first decade after retirement. While the compounded losses continue and increase in the later years, the impact of feelings of loss may be felt first in the 65-75 age period. Loss of mates, brothers and sisters, elderly parents, coworkers, lifetime friends becomes noticeable and has to be dealt with emotionally. Grief and loss of people, position, self-definition, and the recognition and admission of certain physiological changes all impact the young old person. The healthy, well functioning cope with these changes, as they have with other stresses and transitions throughout their life, but they may find that this is a time where they turn for counselling to the mental health professionals. The need for skilled understanding is crucial at this time, and particularly focused on current functioning and the reality of dramatic changes in the person's environment or life-space and life style. There tends to be a high rate of depression at this period which may be treated psychologically or pharmacologically or both. But this is a time when the social worker needs to be particularly sensitive to the total environment and personal/psychological conditions of the person and the family.

One further note about the young old cohort is that many of them have become caretakers of/or responsible for older relatives who have survived to the old old cohort and have become frail and dependent. The young old usually experience a reduction in income (estimated to be about 50 to 70% of their employed income), and sometimes some loss of energy may develop, some chronic illnesses. This is the age period when some noticeable physical and social changes begin to occur, and the person may feel more strongly the sense of losses. At the same time is the added burden or responsibility for older parents. This category of problems began to emerge as an area of concern by social workers and gerontologists in the late 1970's. Social workers are called in to counsel on the burdens and stress of the three and four generation families, to assist families in deciding what older grandparents or parents should do regarding living arrangements.

The majority of young old, in spite of the dramatic changes in their lives, and the impact of the awarenesses of these changes are able to cope, if they have opportunities to find new channels to contribute to society, new challenges to use their talents, and gratifications to replace those they received from their work and family responsibilities.

The Middle Old

The middle old, those between the age of 75 and 84 comprise 28% of the older adult population. People in this age bracket experience more chronic diseases which become debilitating, like arthritis, cardiovascular, respiratory, circulatory disease. These disorders may render a person partially or totally disabled, and dependent. They are physically less active and have more physical decrements than their next younger category. People in this cohort have experienced more stresses through loss of mates, or old-time friends, or relatives of the same generation, and sometimes outlive their children. Women outlive men to a ratio of 178:100 (Brotman).[7]

The people in this cohort tend to be the descendants of a long American past and some are the offspring of the early waves of immigrants from Europe and Asia. Some of these people also came to the U.S. as young adults, and worked in heavy industry, agriculture and domestic work. In this population are many black people whose parents were slaves, or who moved from rural America to the urban areas, and who were the first of their families to earn an independent living, and establish a free life. Social and geographical mobility characterize this population, and although many of them remain in the locale of their growing up, or young adult years, many others have migrated from one section of the country to another. The first major wave of people who moved to the Sunbelt from the Northeast and Middle West were people now in the 75 to 85 age cohort. Retirement communities, begun in the 1950's in Florida, Arizona and Southern California and established by trade unions, religious groups, business and professional associations, lodges and fraternities, attracted these people who felt they were avoiding becoming burdens to their children. These people created surrogate families or pseudofamilies and nonmarital living arrangements to substitute for the families they had left behind, or the mates and peers they had lost. As they reach their late 70's and early 80's, they have become more aware of being survivors and many have chosen communal living in long term care, partial or total care facilities. Others have moved to be near or with their children, as they have reached their later years.

The physiological changes of aging become even more apparent in this 7th and 8th decade of life in the slowing of pace, modification of the senses, particularly eyesight and hearing, the loss of mobility through more difficulties in balance, and less capacity or security in driving. While these decrements are not true for all 75 to 85-year-old people, the occurrence is more frequent. For many people the loss of the capacity to drive through sight impairment, or slowing response time, and judgment of spatial relationships has a negative impact. The person who has to give up driving feels not only loss of status, but also may experience isolation, and become more dependent on others. The decrease of mobility combined with the smaller circle of associations with other survivors, sometimes combined with moving to a new community may result in an isolation, withdrawal into self, and sometimes depression, even disorientation and pseudo senility. This kind of isolation is not true for all people over 70, nor for all people who give up driving, but it is a more apparent problem as a person enters the later years.

Social workers who have an understanding that people are going through natural developmental and decremental processes may be able to help. They can assist the older person who is beginning to worry about himself or herself with some anxiety about the future. They also may assist the relatives of these older people who may be reinforcing these feelings by attempting to make parents more dependent or making decisions for them without involving them. The social worker can also help other professionals who may be called in to assist these older adults, to understand and maximize the strengths and the potentials for self-management, rather than taking independence away. Financial advisors, lawyers, physicians, psychiatrists as well as families, may need the insight which the social worker can offer, of the total person within the particular environment. Every effort to provide the older person with as much control and independence as possible in decision making and self-management will strengthen the integrity of the person.

While we have spoken of some of the decrements of this cohort, it should be remembered that many people in their late 70's and 80's manage very well. More than a quarter of the well elderly, 29% of them, are in the 75-85 year category. Some of the most creative work of civilization has come from people in their 70's and 80's, as has some of the world's great thought and political leadership. More people who reach their 80's every day are remaining physically and socially active, especially as succeeding generations reach old age in better health, are better educated, more active and more involved, and given the opportunities better able to function independently. There is probably greater diversity among 75 to 85 years olds, because of the noticeably different rates of changes of each individual. They have had longer to be different from each other.

The Old Old Population

The *old old population,* those 85 to 95 are also increasing in number, as more people are living longer, but they represent only 8.4% of the older population. The preponderance of this population is frail, dependent, and suffering from more disabilities and chronic diseases. A few are in the well elderly category, going about their daily routines, living alone or with families, driving and managing as always. Those who have survived well in this age category may be particularly strong. Women outlive men on a ratio of 224:100 (Brotman, 1980), making a preponderance of women, mostly widows in this age category. Very few of this population are employed, though some of them work, especially in creative work, or independent activities. Mobility tends to be greatly limited, and involvement decreased. Those who have had reason or have made the effort to be involved with younger persons may continue to have relationships, but a majority of people in their late 80's and 90's have survived their old friends, peers, relatives, mates, and frequently their children and life time associates. The tendency toward social isolation becomes even greater for this cohort, as they have more physical decrements and are more vulnerable to disabling diseases, accidents and environmental impacts. The incidence of mental disorders from physical changes are also greater in this period. Although only 4 to 5% of older people ever develop senility, a larger proportion of the population, perhaps as much as 10-15% of this very old population may show evidences of brain disorders or senility (Butler, 1980).[8]

A phenomenon referred to as "crossing over" occurs within this cohort population, in that blacks who generally have a shorter life span than persons of other races, tend to outnumber the population of whites in the over 80 category. According to Jackson (1980),[9] blacks who survive to over 80, tend to outlive other populations. The only speculative explanation for this phenomenon is that those who have survived the hardships of minority status throughout a lifetime of great transitions, have the stamina to outlive others once they reach a very old age.

LIFE EXPECTANCY

The life span or life expectancy of most species of animals remains almost constant. For humans the span is approximately 110 to 120 years, according to biologists and geneticists (Woodruff, 1973).[10] That few people have lived that long is due not to their life expectancy but to the risks of the human society, exposure to diseases, engagement in activities that shorten the life, such as smoking or abuse of drugs or alcohol, or the risks of the environment, poor air, accidents, pressures and tensions of the workplace and interpersonal relationships. That many more people could live to be 100 and many more do each year, is a well established fact. If the pattern continues to exist that old age begins in the 60's, and that people beyond 65 may not continue to be productive in the workplace, or have few functional roles in their families, or are not given leadership roles in the community, people who live to their 80's, 90's and 100's will be relegated to a period of 30, 40 or 50 years of old age in obsolescence. There is a tendency to lump this entire age period into one set of characteristics called "old age." For no other age span have the social or behavioral sciences done this. Infancy, early childhood, later childhood, adolescence, young adulthood, middle age each cover a shorter period of time ranging from 3 or 4 years to a decade. The physiological changes, psychological changes, social experiences and personal characteristics of people beyond early 60's are as dramatic in 5 to 10 year age spans as they are earlier in life. Yet they have not so far been distinguished in the same way, nor given specific labels or names. The reasons are explainable. Until recently, well functioning, healthy people in any great numbers have not been studied longitudinally from ages 60 to 100. Secondly the research of any significance has only begun to emerge to show physiological and psychological changes at different older adult age stages. And third there is a very wide variation in the rates of changes of those whose chronological age is similar. Variations include heredity, immunity, lifestyles and patterns, health histories, access to the resources of the society to help avert diseases and accidents and exposure to external risks. Furthermore, the quality of life for the very old has not necessarily supported a motivation toward seeking greater personal fulfillment in the later years except for the wealthy, or those with strong multigenerational family ties and traditions, or for those in creative or professional occupations where there was the possibility for pursuing a career throughout one's life. What is needed then, is a different perspective on aging, a corrected vision and view which will effect services and the way older adults are involved in their own futures.

DEFINITIONS OF AGING

Birren (1980)[11] has noted that aging may be seen as (a) chronological, by years and passage of time, (b) physiological by the physical changes that occur in one's body functions and systems and physical features, (c) psychological or the mental capacities and personality changes over time, and that these three types of aging occur differently for different individuals. Actually there is also social aging—a process that occurs in one's social and personal relationships. Social aging is in part due to a person's physical and psychological capacities which prolong or limit interactions with others. In part, social aging is due to self-expectation for continued relationships. Social aging is also associated to the socialization process throughout life that has conditioned one to expect certain roles and life patterns in old age, and in part to respond to society or the environmental factors that pressure these responses. These environmental factors would include social policies regarding work and retirement, employment opportunities, economic supports, housing and living style, the nature of relationships, the loss of peers through death or mobility, and the actual economics of financial resources available to the person through any means.

There are so many variations in individuals as they age in each of these aspects of the aging process that it is difficult to draw generalizations about age difference. But of course in many ways the same may be said about adolescence, young adulthood and middle age. The older population has had longer to become different from each other. Furthermore as we have noted, social history for each cohort of aging has been very different with the technological changes and the social revolutions which have occurred over the past 100 years, particularly in American life. Therefore among the older population there are also regional, ethnic, racial, socioeconomic as well as sex differences.

Most probably the research exists that would make possible some clear distinctions of categories of the aging population. Yet traditional references still treat old age as one single life period from 60 or 65 until 90 or 100. Thus categories seem to be descriptive: the well elderly and the frail and dependent elderly, the institutionalized elderly or the elderly living in the community. And the labels attached are not definitive, but may be derogative, such as senior citizens, older adults, senior adults, golden agers, elderly, geronts, old codgers, old maids, old men and women. The derogation may not be so much in the label as in the social connotations that old is lesser, or obsolete, or useless. This connotation developed within a social milieu that has emphasized growth, expansion, productivity, vigor, youth and active survival, rather than traditions, history, heritage and vintage. While this attitude may be changing, especially as the population ages, there is as yet no major thrust in the total society toward distinguishing the various phases and aspects of old age.

Suffice to say there exists within the population of old age now, close to 12 to 15% of the total population of the nation with vast differences and variations which need to be viewed and understood, not only by those working with them, but by the general population; those who are old and those who live with them.

SOCIAL WORK PRACTICE WITH THE WELL ELDERLY

Aging is a natural condition of living, a normal growth process over the life span in the person effecting all aspects of life; physical, mental, emotional and social, including changes in patterns of relationship in families, work, and community. Old age includes the potential for incremental growth and change as well as the potential for decremental change and losses. Frequently old age has been seen by social workers and others in the human services professions as a period of breakdown, a problem time of sickness, deterioration, and the end of life. These misconceptions about old age have developed from the experience of many professionals who see only the oldest adults, or those who are ill and frail, who have come to clinics, long-term care facilities or old age homes. Yet there are social and personal needs of the well elderly for which social workers can be well prepared to assist.

Social workers can become engaged with the well older adults who have many talents, wisdom and energy to be channeled into new careers, working with their peers, as counsellors, friendly visitors, volunteers, trainers, teaching assistants, surrogate families, as well as policymakers, public administrators or governmental assistants. Social workers need to learn how to work with talented and experienced older adults without feeling threatened by the knowledge, status, expertise or age brought by the seniors. At the same time role definition and time limitations and demands need to be spelled out carefully to establish constructive contributions, each to the other. Most older adults who are well and have considerable energy, also have fairly clear notions about what kinds of responsibilities they wish to take and how much energy they have to invest. Some of them may lack direction, because they have not thought about their futures. Some older adults who have retired and have some sense of loss of direction may express their anxiety through expressions of lack of the self confidence which they have had in previous life experiences, or an overassertive stance to prove to themselves and others that they are adequate. The sensitive social worker will understand where such behavior originates and will be neither threatened nor antagonized by it. They will encourage the person to engage in appropriate activity. Just as the adolescent who faces emotions, physical responses, and social demands that are different from his previous life experiences, as he moves through the physical and emotional changes of puberty and therefore needs help in finding himself and takes on new and adaptive behaviors, so some older people who experience physical changes, energy changes, modification in what have been previous life roles and relationships, must have some understanding and guidance to relocate themselves in their new life space as they age.

Many older adults have been so busy throughout life on an externally prescribed schedule or plan of life, determined by the demands of their jobs, their families, their social activities, that they find themselves at a loss at retirement, or when these demands taper off. They have to learn to set their own schedules, their pace, their programs, and become more self-directing. The period of transition into retirement is therefore a very difficult transition point for these people during which they need a variety of kinds of support. There is evidence of increased stress and the psychosomatic symptoms of stress, higher incidence of illness, depression and dramatic behavioral changes during this period for many people. Sometimes longtime marriages or other kinds of relationships break up at this time. Social workers could well develop more expertise in industrial social work in preretirement planning and counselling, and post-retirement family and marital counselling, as well as in developing programs of transition for people to find new roles and responsibilities as they retire. Sometimes the period of stress is not immediate upon retirement, when there is a feeling of relief from the regularity of the schedule, and the pressures of responsibilities. Many people engage in activities which they have delayed through their working years and schedule activities, travel, volunteer work and recreation. Generally, however, during the first five years of retirement there develops a period of stress, when the person may seek help in sorting out mixed emotions about retirement, or may develop physical or emotional symptoms of stress. The skilled and perceptive social worker can be helpful in providing appropriate assessment, support, guidance, direction and counsel.

The longer people live, the more capable they are of coping with the changes that occur in their environment. While the stresses of retirement, of role changes, of the loss of peers, relatives and friends through death or mobility to other places, may produce some depression and need for counsel, most older adults cope with their transitions, their illnesses and losses and move on. They acquire a perspective, wisdom and experience, which is a rich resource for the sociocultural milieu. They have spent their lives adapting to some of the most dramatic technological, social and cultural changes in the world's history. They have experienced wars, depressions, industrial development, the advent of radio, television, the automobile and the growth of cities with centralization of urban services, and decentralization to suburbia. They have experienced the sexual revolution, and the change of traditional views of the family with changing roles for children, women and men in society. They have witnessed the birth of rapid communication and transmittal of information on a global basis, computerization and rapidly changing financial management systems, uses of tapes, video tapes and other electronic means for recall and communications, and the possibility of space colonization. These changes over a lifetime of anyone over the age of sixty have necessitated adaptations, changes, growth and flexibility, not only in life style, but in custom and culture, including modifications in values, beliefs, ways of living and perspective and knowledge. They have also experienced feelings about obsolescence of things, people and relationships. In addition, the change to the general availability and accessibility of the arts and education have made possible a change in the cultural experience and outlook of many people and their use of education as a means of adaptation. The longer a person has lived, the more drastic and dramatic the changes are and have been. The availability and variety of foods and resources, taken for granted by younger people who have always seen them around and have had them or aspired to have them, continues to be a source of amazement to many older people who lived through a period of greater simplicity and even lack of resources in their early years, and during wars and depression. But having adapted to these changes, the older population has acquired a habit of adapting to change, expecting the unexpected, and while sometimes resisting change or fighting it, ultimately adopting and adapting to the dynamic waves of social and cultural modifications.

Most older people, however, have difficulty with the concept of planned obsolescence, discarding of things, ideas, or relationships when they have become dysfunctional or worn out. Many people in their 60's, 70's and 80's lived with poor relationships rather than discarding unhappy or difficult marriages, conflicts with relatives, friends or neighbors. Many are resistant to the idea of using a counsellor to change things. The idea, therefore, of late life separations, leaving of difficult situations or the use of counsellors, especially for people in their 80's and older, takes considerable shifting of perspective, values and beliefs. For many in the middle classes and even some in lower economic populations, to resort to the use of a "welfare system" for programs, senior centers, nutrition programs, counselling, economic support or other programs and services may be a reflection of weakness, failure, incapacity, indicating loss of integrity and self-sufficiency. The American work ethic has even permeated some of the population which has lived close to the margin of partial employment, or survived on welfare assistance through a large part of life.

From the standpoint of planning for the future and thinking about the resources needed by older people, one definitive fact is available. Everyone who will reach 65 by 2030 has already been born. Considering current research and advancement in medical treatment for dealing with chronic and catastrophic diseases, psychological procedures for stress reduction and social programs for working on family relations and life styles, there will continue to be a prolonged life span for people of each succeeding generation. More people will live longer barring a war or major physical catastrophe or uncontrolled epidemic. Even in the cohorts where there have been reduced numbers of children, it can be predicted that more people will live longer with an even higher survivorship.

As more people grow older there is and will be a continuing need to develop more social programs and services which increase the opportunities for the well elderly, who make up the majority of people over 65. Although social services, quite appropriately have tended to focus on remedial needs, care for the frail, dependent, deteriorated, ill elderly who are in need of care, protection and supportive programs, it should be remembered that this population comprises approximately 5 to 20% of the people 65 and older. Social work professionals have within their knowledge, skill, values and philosophy, the history, tradition and capability to develop and manage programs and services which can provide needed opportunity for adequate functioning and contribution of the well older adults of all ages from 60 to 90. There are many resources available for the development and management of programs with older adults. The social work profession and social welfare services have only scratched the surface of the contribution which could be made through direct clinical services, community services and social policy and planning with the aging.

It has been suggested that while social service programs for the frail dependent and ill older people have been more or less adequately handled by social workers, who can move in on problems, pathology and defined social needs, the preventive, social programs have been less well handled. In part this may be due to the prevalence in the past of a "sickness" model of aging, viewing old age as a breakdown, decremental losses and the end of life, rather than a growth model of old age as a series of stages of life transitions and changes with the potential for growth even when decrements exist. The stereotypes of old age prevalent in the wider culture have permeated all professions including social work, to the extent that they have prevented the most adequate use of knowledge and skill. The stereotypes have hindered the development of creative, imaginative new programs to provide greater opportunities for participation of people in their later years. Social work as a profession has the knowledge that can be applied to the creation of programs that will sustain and support older persons within the mainstream of their families, their communities, the workplace and the marketplace to ensure the use of their resources and contributions, maintain their feelings of adequacy and self-esteem, and define appropriate roles and functions with them as an integral segment of society. While social workers and social welfare services alone cannot modify society or create these new opportunities, they can, in collaboration with education, the political structure, health system, religious system, business and industry, make some changes in attitudes about the opportunities for older adults. They can eliminate the stereotypes and misconceptions from the culture of social work and social welfare, and remove institutional ageism where it exists within the profession.

STEREOTYPES OF AGING

Stereotypically, old age is seen as the end of the line, a period of increased decrements and a period of withdrawal from society. This perception of aging is held by the general public, which includes professionals working with people, and especially people in their younger years. But it is also held especially by people reaching their 60's who have been socialized to believe that life after middle age—the 40's and the 50's—is all downhill, a time to withdraw from activity and responsibility, and a time to question one's capacity, ability, creativity or contribution to society. In part this attitude towards aging has developed in a culture that measures a person by productivity, working on a job, producing a family, creating new ideas in the arts, literature, sciences, maintaining a household, and taking community responsibility and/or organizational leadership. These values regarding a person's role in society in the United States are held in each of the socioeconomic levels, though their manifestation differs with differing life styles. When old age has been associated with nonwork, increased dependency, slackening responsibility and a series of physical, psychological and social losses, the perception of aging has taken negative connotations to be avoided, feared, rejected and worried about. This is true for the people facing old age who may fear a process they cannot stop or control, and for younger persons who respond by avoiding and rejecting those who have arrived at and are living through old age.

It is therefore sometimes viewed with surprise that people in their 60's, 70's, or 80's continue to be active, involved, productive members of society, so long as they have or make the opportunities to do so. People who are involved and productive and maintain good health habits, short of some sort of physical or social accident, disease, or catastrophic illness, who come from a strong heredity, or who have had education or economics that are resources for good health and emotional maintenance, reach their later years with considerable vigor and the capacity to maintain a full life.

There has been a rapid rise in the number of people who are

reaching their later years. In the past 80 years, the average life expectancy has risen from 47.3 in 1900 to approximately 73.3 in 1980. This increase is due not so much to care in the later years, as to advancement in health and mental health care throughout the life cycle (particularly in childhood and youth); in developing immunity to certain diseases; in the management of circulatory and respiratory diseases, and cancer; in better economic resources and community resources; improved nutrition; and to some degree better stress management, and education that helps people to find the resources they need. All are causes of the increase in life expectancy. There are however, still populations where less resources are available. Older people of some of the ethnic populations have not had the advantages that provide pensions, social security, health resources, and access to various community resources. These populations at risk are in need of further social research and social work intervention to provide more adequate services.

The total range of social work resources from prevention to therapeutic, from partial to total care, from individual counselling to case management of varied resources, is needed within the social welfare services for the normal aging and their families. These areas will be covered by the chapters that follow.

REFERENCES

1. Brotman, H., Every Ninth American, Report to the Senate, Special committee on Aging, U.S. Govt. Printing Office, Washington, D.C., 1980.
2. Neugarten, Bernice L., Age Groups in American Society and the Rise of the Young Old, *Annals of American Academy of Sciences,* Sept. 1974.
3. Cain, Leonard, Age Status and generational phenomenon. The new old people in contemporary America, *Gerontologist,* 1980.
4. McConnell, S.R., Alternative Work Patterns for an Aging Work Force in Ragan, P. (ed) *Work and Retirement, Policy Issues,* Los Angeles Andrus Gerontology Center, U.S.C., 1978.
5. Brotman, H. op. cit.
6. Ibid.
7. Ibid.
8. Butler, Robert & Lewis, Myrna, *Aging and Mental Health,* 3rd ed., St. Louis, C.V. Mosby Co., 1982.
9. Jackson, Jacqueline J., *Ethnic Minorities and Aging,* Belmont, Ca., Wadsworth Press, 1980.
10. Woodruff, Diane, *Can You Live to be 100?,* N.Y., New American Library Inc., 1977.
11. Birren, James & Renner, Jayne, Concepts and Issues of Mental Health and Aging in Birren, J. & Sloane, R. (eds) *Handbook of Mental Health and Aging,* Englewood Cliffs, N.J., Prentice Hall, 1980.

ADDITIONAL READINGS

Beaver, Marion L., Prevention, the Well Elderly and Social Casework. Univ. of Pittsburgh, paper delivered at AGHE conference, Cincinnati, 1981. Unpublished.

Hartford, Margaret. The Use of Group Methods for Work with the Aged in Birren, J. & Sloane, B. (eds) *Handbook of Mental Health and Aging.* Englewood Cliffs, N.J., Prentice Hall, 1980, pp. 806-820.

Hartford, Margaret E., The Strength of the Well Elderly in Davis, R. (ed) *Aging Prospects and Issues.* Andrus Gerontology Center, U.S.C., Lexington Press, 1981, pp. 160-174.

Hartford, Margaret E., The uses of groups with relatives of frail and dependent elderly, *Gerontologist,* Oct., 1982.

National Institute on Aging, Special Report on Aging, 1980. U.S. Dept. of Health & Human Services, P.H.S., N.I.H. & N.I.A., Publications #80-2135, Aug. 1980, Washington, D.C.

United States Dept. of Commerce, Bureau of Census, Social and Economic Characteristics of the Older Population. Special Studies Series, 1978, pp 23-85.

Weg, Ruth B., *The Aged, Who, Where, How Well.* Leonard Davis School of Gerontology, University of Southern California, Los Angeles, Ca., 1981.

Chapter IV

Social Work Practice
With the Aged and Their Families:
A Systems Approach

Charlotte Kirschner

More than twenty years ago, gerontologists began to call attention
to the importance of families in the lives of the elderly.[1] It is by now
an established fact that the family is the primary social support
system for individuals who need help with the normal dependencies
of aging. Indeed, the mental health of older people is closely linked
to their family relations.[2] It is also true that the younger generation
needs and wants good relationships with its elders. An interactional
and reciprocal process among family members occurs at any age.[3]
Nathan Ackerman, a pioneer in the study of family dynamics,
pointed out that a crisis in the life of one member of a family may
have pervasive and far-reaching effects on the mental health of the
others.[4] Developing skills for treating families in later life has therefore become a major challenge to the helping professions, given the
rapidly growing numbers of elderly in our population. It is the thesis
of this paper that gerontological social workers should be familiar
with the theory and practice of family therapy and use this form of
treatment, when appropriate, to help their clients face the crisis of
aging.

Gerontological research has shown that the vast majority of older
Americans have living relatives and are in contact with them frequently; tend to live near their adult children; exchange mutual aid;
and report concern and positive feelings for each other.[5] Adult children have been found to be intensely involved in helping their
parents cope with a wide range of problems,[6] and to provide extensive assistance to them at substantial sacrifice and strain.[7]

55

STRESS OF FAMILY CAREGIVING

The stresses and strains inherent in family relationships in later life have been well documented.[8] One source of stress can be the result of the conflict between two highly valued American traditions, family loyalty and individualism, especially when the transitional tasks of the family do not mesh with the transitional tasks of individual members.[9] According to Erik Erikson, any transitional period in life carries with it specific developmental tasks which must be completed.[10] But families have life cycles of their own, and their emotional energies are usually invested elsewhere when an aging parent needs help. Adult children are developing careers or coping with problems of menopause and retirement; grandchildren are dealing with adolescence or new marriages; great-grandchildren are being born, creating four and five generation families. The adult son or daughter, caught in the middle, feels the strain. More often it is the daughter[11] who faces meeting the publisher's deadline for the article she is writing, taking her ailing mother to the doctor, and watching her teenager perform in the school play, sometimes all on the same day! In an extreme case, the parent can be neglected if the family is otherwise involved.

Case Example. Mrs. T. called the social worker for advice about getting a companion for her mother, age 79, who lived alone and was showing evidence of senile dementia. She had severe memory loss, was suspicious of everyone, and had been neglecting herself and her home. On further questioning it was learned that she had recently discharged her housekeeper who had been with her for 30 years, and had refused to keep anyone her daughter hired. The landlord was threatening to evict her because she had repeatedly let the bathtub run over, causing a flood and damage to her apartment and the one below. The social worker arranged to meet the daughter and son-in-law at the mother's home.

The social worker found an extremely deteriorated situation. The mother was dressed in a thin, sleeveless summer dress although it was winter and there was snow on the ground. Dishes on the dining room table were encrusted with stale food. The mother screamed at the worker, ordering her to leave. A geriatric psychiatrist and nurse were recommended who would make a home visit and help the family bring the mother to a private hospital where she could be admitted for an evaluation and further planning.

When asked how long this condition had been going on, the daughter guiltily explained that it had been several months, but she and her husband had not wanted to do anything until after their daughter's wedding, which had just taken place. They had managed to clean mother up and get her to the wedding so the new in-laws would not know the family secret.

Stress is also felt by families who are torn between a desire to take care of parents and a recognition that old people should maintain their independence for as long as possible. Fears of illness and death, and the pain of watching a loved parent deteriorate, add to the burdens felt by families at this stage of life. In the case of an adult child who may not have experienced good parenting, there can be anger and resentment at being called upon to help, with the accompanying guilt at not wanting to help.

The greatest source of stress is guilt for seemingly never fulfilling one's obligation to a parent no matter how hard one tries. The extent of one's sense of obligation can be determined internally through an adult child's emotional makeup, and his or her need for love and recognition, or it can be externally imposed by a parent in the form of implicit, unexpressed expectations carried over from one generation to another. Boszormenyi-Nagy and Spark have described a transgenerational bookkeeping system with invisible accounts in which loyalty owed to a parent becomes a debt that can never be repaid.[12] Small wonder that many sons and daughters are never liberated from a sense of guilt at not being able to do for their aging parents as much as was done for them when they were young.[13]

Gerontologists, sensitive to these stresses and strains on families, have increasingly been turning their attention to working for programs and policies designed to relieve families of some of the practical and psychological burdens they carry in later life. The 33rd Annual Scientific Meeting of the Gerontological Society of America in November 1980 was devoted to the theme, "Families of the Aged." One of the highlights of that meeting was a hearing conducted by the Select Committee on Aging of the House of Representatives of the U.S. Congress, at which experts testified on behalf of the needs of families. The important role played by the families of the aged had previously come to lawmakers' attention in the report to the Congress by the Comptroller General of the U.S. on December 30, 1977, in which it was pointed out that families were the chief providers of care to the infirm elderly.[14]

FAMILY SERVICES

With this increasing focus on the needs of families in later life, funding has been made available and programs have been developed on behalf of families of the aged in many locations around the country. Demonstration projects, conferences, group meetings, and training programs are educating families on the aging process and helping them cope with the emotional impact that an aging parent has on the rest of the family. It is possible to replicate many of these programs by sending for their manuals.[15] Silverstone and Hyman's guidebook, which helps adult children deal with the emotional, physical, and financial problems of aging parents, is in its second edition, testifying to the great need of modern families for such information.[16]

Yet the concept of family treatment has not had a very great impact on the field of gerontology. Family therapy has caught the interest of the helping professions and the general public to such a degree that daily newspapers and popular magazines are featuring articles on the subject. But, with a few exceptions,[17] family therapists use this modality only when a young child is the "identified patient." Gerontologists, for the most part, view family counseling as a corollary to the treatment of the aged person, instead of seeing the aged person *and* his or her family as the unit of attention. Aged persons should not be treated in isolation, but should be seen as participants in a total family system.

FAMILY AS A SYSTEM

Family therapy is a logical outgrowth of the ecological movement, which emphasizes the relation between organisms and their environments and the adaptive process by which they achieve a good fit. The ecological movement and family therapy are both based on the concept of the system and the consciousness of the interdependence of life and the conditions that support it.[18] Viewing the family as a system recognizes that family members are related by means of an organizational structure with boundaries, rules and regulations, and a power hierarchy, which enable them to carry out their functions. At different periods of development the family is required to adapt to changing circumstances and take on new functions by restructuring its organization.[19] A young couple, leaving its family of origin, creates its own new family system with its unique characteristics while still maintaining its ties to the parental generation. Changes occur over time as children are born and grow to maturity. An open system accommodates to these changes as developmental milestones occur both in the children and in the parents. As this young couple grows older, its maturing children in turn move away, marry, and create new families, and again the system changes. Subsystems are formed, each with their own unique organization consisting of boundaries, rules, power structures, and sets of relationships. Each extended family now finds a new equilibrium among the subsystems, which enables it to maintain intergenerational relationships during this transitional phase.

In the next phase of life the crisis of aging can confront a family with a new set of demands in the form of the dependency needs of a parent. The system that maintained family equilibrium at a distance may become dysfunctional at a time of developmental change and accompanying stress. A changed system with a new organization must be created to accommodate to the crisis. This requires a renegotiation of boundaries, a new distribution of functions, and a change in leadership. Authority usually shifts from the aged parents to the middle-aged children or to one designated middle-aged child.

Most families weather the crisis of aging without seeking professional help. Adult children who have achieved what Margaret Blenkner called "filial maturity" are able to free themselves of their childhood roles, achieve the capacity to be depended upon, and assume the responsibilities that the new situation demands.[20] They are able spontaneously to form a new system organized around a mutual aid network to meet the changing needs of the aging parent.

Case Example. When Mr. J., a 74-year-old widower, was ready to be discharged from the hospital after hip replacement surgery, his four adult children held a family conference at his bedside. Knowing he wanted to return to his own home rather than stay with any one of them, they made a plan for the immediate future. Amy's children were going to camp for the summer. Since she was divorced and would have no one at home, she agreed to move in with Dad for a few weeks until he got on his feet again. Louise, who lived nearby and was a marvelous cook, would prepare several casseroles each week and put them in Dad's freezer for Amy to heat and serve. John, a physical fitness buff, would come two evenings a week after work to help Dad continue the exercises that had been started on the rehabilitation unit. Frank, who lived out of town and had come in for the conference, invited Dad to spend two weeks at his house as soon as he was able to get around a little better. With everyone cooperating, Mr. J. and his family managed to set up a system which saw him through his convalescence.

Other families need help in solving this developmental problem, and a systems orientation is a useful tool for the gerontological social worker. Facing a crisis with an aging parent, family members may be in fixed positions which do not accommodate change, and therefore they may become immobilized. An authoritarian father may still inappropriately rule the family from his bed in the hospital, instead of allowing the power structure to shift to his perfectly competent children; feuding brothers and sisters may be unable to agree to a new distribution of functions in order to come to the aid of a parent; a mother may refuse to accept the help she needs from her adult children, thus trapping them in a guilt-inducing system which blocks all attempts at reciprocity. These are examples of closed systems in which all efforts are nullified through endless repetition of ineffective, stereotyped responses. The therapeutic task is to open the system so it can change in response to changing conditions.[21]

SOCIAL WORK INTERVENTION

(A). With the Family

The social worker can observe the system in operation by bringing the family together—aging parents, adult children and their spouses, even grandchildren when they are closely involved with their grandparents. The very act of assembling the family can sometimes open the system to change. An initial interview with the entire family, preferably in the home, will enable the social worker "to evaluate individual psychodynamics, family interaction, living arrangements, neighborhood supports, and financial status. . . [and] will help the social worker decide where intervention is likely to be most effective in order to help the aging parent and to bring the family to the point where it can make realistic decisions about meeting his or her needs."[22] The choice of intervention will depend on the worker's observation of whether dysfunctional patterns within the family system or within the larger environment are creating the current imbalance. Often families only need to be educated about the availability of community resources and the rights of their aged parents to financial assistance, and they can then manage very well.

There are always greater demands on the social worker when a family is congregated in his or her office, because of the multiple impact of the group and the "feelings which are aroused in everybody when family matters and issues are expressed and played out."[22] The worker may think the elderly parent is too fragile to be exposed to the dynamics of family interaction, when, in fact, the parent has been exposed to it all his life and has usually had a hand in creating it and controlling it. Social workers may be struggling with their own family relationship difficulties and therefore experience stress when they meet similar situations in their clients.[23] Workers must overcome their own anxieties about family involvement, or, at least, separate their anxieties from those of their clients, before they can intervene successfully with families.

Case Example. Janet S. joined the social service department of a nursing home when she completed her professional education. Her grandmother had lived with the family while Janet was growing up, and she and Janet had been very close. Janet was therefore well prepared for work with the aged, and she enjoyed a good relationship with her clients.

However, when the middle aged daughter of one of the residents had some complaint about the food, Janet showed a lack of sensitivity in speaking to her, and the woman asked to see the director.

Discussing this in supervision, Janet realized the incident reminded her of a similar situation that had often occurred at home. This resident's middle aged daughter reminded Janet of her own mother, and conflicts they had experienced with each other about Grandma were rekindled for Janet, making it difficult for her to maintain her professional composure in the presence of her client's family. When she was able to separate her own family problems from those of her clients, Janet was able to be more helpful to the adult children of the nursing home residents.

Social workers may share the misgiving of a well known geriatric psychiatrist that family sessions "may be opening not a dialogue but a can of worms. . . [in terms of] the intensity of. . . feelings, the ramifications arising from long past history, and the recrudescence. . . of childhood difficulties.''[24] To avoid the pitfalls inherent in such a psychoanalytical approach, the social worker should view the family as a system and deal only with the here and now. By concentrating on the present problem the family can be helped to reorganize around a solution to the immediate crisis.[25] Family therapy can also heal relationships and build bridges between the generations, and this is often the fortunate outcome of crisis resolution, but an introspective, uncovering type of treatment requires a different contract between worker and client. Social workers must try to avoid opening old wounds. Family sessions should be used to validate and interpret the different positions of family members, help them listen to and really hear one another, and clear up myths and misunderstandings. Families must be guided through the present reality to a resolution of the aging parents' crisis. The worker is not responsible for finding solutions. The task is to present the options, remove the obstacles to constructive communication, block dysfunctional interaction, and create an atmosphere in which family members can work together toward finding their own solutions.

Social workers meet clients in a variety of settings where they have the opportunity to intervene in the problems of the extended family at different developmental stages. The function of a particular agency will usually define the extent of the social worker's involvement with clients' families, and some agency workers will therefore be limited in the scope of their interventions. If family treatment is indicated, and the agency cannot provide it, the family should be referred elsewhere. The case examples given here are taken from a private, fee for service consultation center for aged persons and their families, and while private practice offers the luxury of a broader field of action, the principles are applicable to other settings as well.

A systems orientation to working with families of the aged does not dictate that the entire family must always be seen together, although this is highly recommended, especially as a diagnostic tool.[26] The social worker may choose to work with one or another subsystem, always thinking of the effects of the professional intervention on the total family system: ''. . . practitioners. . . need to have a choice of intervention at their disposal and. . . the type of intervention should be determined by a particular family's life phase, structure, and specific needs.''[27]

(B). With Elderly Couples

The life phase of the so-called "empty nest" leaves the older couple alone again. The adult children, if there have been children, leave the family of origin to create new families or new lifestyles. Many couples report that marriage is better than ever at this phase of life, with more privacy and less family responsibility.[28] For others, however, illness or disability shifts the balance in the relationship between the spouses and marriage in late life may be "filled with shared heightened anxiety, interpersonal difficulties and economic strains."[29] Getzel, in describing an interventive model for work with aging couples, points out the effect on the total family system of a crisis in their lives. "The balance of caregiving demands between spouses varies in intensity as do the capacities of spouses to fulfill demands placed on them. The capacities of spouses to meet these reciprocal demands have significant implications for elderly couples' children, siblings, other relatives and friends who may be called on to fill gaps."[30] The varied needs of older couples who have remained together for a lifetime have been well illustrated in Getzel's study. The social work task in meeting these needs includes exploring the stresses of caregiving, helping the caring spouse recognize the partner's condition, facilitating communication, and encouraging life review and reconciliation of feelings, all leading to an acceptance of the realistic options for care which are open to the couple.

Remarried couples are especially vulnerable to the crisis of aging, and their difficulties can reverberate upon an extremely complicated family network with multiple branches and no history of shared experiences to fall back on at a time of stress. In later life, illness and disability often strike a blow at a remarried couple from which the relationship cannot recover.

Case Example. Mr. and Mrs. V., age 81 and 76, had been married for three years when he had a stroke which left him with garbled speech, an inability to use his right hand, and increasing irritability. Mrs. V. had been left a widow after 45 years of marriage, and had married Mr. V., a widower and a successful businessman, for companionship and financial security. Within the first six months, however, she had considered divorce, because his disposition was difficult, and vastly different from that of her first husband. She thought it would be better to be married than to be lonely, and so she decided to remain with Mr. V.

After his stroke, her two adult children urged her to place him in a nursing home, while his children pressured her to bring him home from the hospital. She could not decide what to do, and became immobilized by anxiety and depression.

Her oldest son consulted the social worker, who suggested a family meeting including both sets of adult children. After two family sessions and three individual sessions with Mrs. V., a compromise was worked out whereby she would bring Mr. V. home from the hospital and enroll him three days a week in a Day Hospital for the aged, where he would receive speech therapy and physiotherapy. With his funds going for rehabilitation, Mrs. V. realized she would have neither companionship nor financial security, and once again she thought about divorce. She decided to wait six months and then review her options.

(C). With the Widowed

Widowhood in old age is well known to create problems in the family system, drawing adult children back into the parental orbit under changed circumstances. Family sessions can clear the air, help dispel myths and unrealistic expectations, and move the family toward helpful planning for the bereaved spouse.

Case Example. When Mrs. E. was left a widow at age 81, her two adult children and their families were prepared for her grief, but they were very much surprised when they realized that she was quite unable to take care of herself. They always had known that Dad had been the more dominant member of the pair, but they had never realized just how much their mother had depended on him. She was fearful of going out, could not shop for food, expected the children to bring her meals, and often spent the day alone, not even getting dressed. She telephoned one or another family member at various times of the day and night, expressing fear that someone was trying to break into her apartment.

Her daughter consulted the social worker, who arranged for a home visit with both adult children and their spouses present. Mrs. E. vetoed every suggestion that was made and was particularly opposed to hiring a companion, although she was well able to afford one. Finally her son asked, with exasperation, what they could do to help. Mrs. E., her lips trembling, asked if she couldn't please move in with one of them? They all looked very uncomfortable, and no one was able to reply. The social worker then asked each one in turn to describe his or her family responsibilities and living arrangements, and it soon became apparent that for one reason or another Mrs. E. could not move in with either family. Everyone realized that Mrs. E. had been clinging to the hope that one of her children would rescue her. She had been afraid to say it, and they had been afraid to hear it.

The presence and skill of the social worker had enabled the family to discuss this emotionally laden subject openly. Once the fantasy of moving in with a child was put to rest, Mrs. E. was able to look realistically at her other options. The social worker saw the family three more times, after which Mrs. E. chose to take a room in a hotel for senior citizens where she made a good adjustment.

Widowhood of an adult child in middle age can create a very special family subsystem composed of a widowed parent and a widowed child. This pair may be an elderly mother and a middle aged son; an elderly father and a middle aged daughter; or widowed parent and widowed child of the same sex. Any one of these combinations can present a problem in maintaining boundaries between the generations, but the daughter left in this position is especially vulnerable to the expectation that she will take care of her father, who may have had no experience in keeping house for himself. Any move she may want to make toward creating a new life for herself may be blocked by the guilt she feels about her unfulfilled obligation to care for her old father.

Case Example. After his wife's death, Mr. R.'s only daughter and son-in-law invited the 84-year-old gentleman to live with them. The son-in-law had lost his own father when he was young, and he was quite attached to his wife's father. His wife was delighted with the arrangement, as they all got along well, and she had less to worry about with her father under her own roof.

Unfortunately, the son-in-law died in a tragic automobile accident, and the daughter, short of funds, was forced to go back to teaching, a profession from which she had taken early retirement. Her father, left alone all day, became depressed. The daughter, herself bereaved, also became depressed and had trouble concentrating on her work. The family physician recommended a consultation with the social worker.

The social worker saw Mr. R. and his daughter in weekly sessions for two months, during which time she helped the pair mourn their losses. Fearing they would stir up too much emotion in each other, they had avoided all mention of the recent deaths of their close relatives. They felt much relief in talking about them, and after a while they were able to talk about the future. The father insisted that his continued presence in his daughter's home was deterring her from making a new life for herself, and he began to investigate other arrangements. The social worker helped him locate an apartment in a special housing project for the elderly. Six months later the daughter called the worker to tell her she was seeing an old friend who had remained a bachelor. She and her friend frequently visited her father who was making his own friends in the housing project. Social work intervention had enabled this pair to maintain an appropriate father-daughter relationship without becoming enmeshed with each other.

(D). With Siblings

Finally, the sibling subsystem can become an area of professional intervention when the parent is too frail to be involved, or when the parents are no longer living, and the aging brothers and sisters are called upon to help one another at periods of crisis.

Case Example. Mrs. N., age 73, called the social worker for help in locating a companion for her sister, Miss F., age 69, who had recently been hospitalized for severe depression and was now home. The sister had never married and was living alone. The hospital social worker had not helped with any plans for home care because, when ready for discharge, the patient felt well enough to manage on her own. A few weeks later, however, she became panicky and called her older sister, Mrs. N., who responded as she had done all her life—that is, she was prepared to take over. The social worker asked if there were any other siblings in the family, and learned that there was another sister and a brother. A family conference was arranged in the worker's office, including the patient, her two sisters and her brother, all over the age of 65.

During the family discussion it became apparent that the patient had experienced a temporary set-back, putting in motion an automatic interaction between the two sisters in which the older one felt obligated to take charge, and the younger one became dependent on her. By helping them to recall similar episodes in the past, the social worker was able to involve all the siblings in a mutual aid system which relieved Mrs. N. of the caretaker role which she had always assumed. More frequent contact with the sister and brother who had been feeling left out enabled Miss F. to continue to care for herself.

CONCLUSION

It is one of social work's basic values to help strengthen family ties. With the current population explosion of the aged in our society, Ethel Shanas' prediction of 1962 is fast coming true: She said then that the problem of aging parents was likely soon to become one of the most pressing of our time.[31] Social workers in the field of aging must meet the challenge of helping the families of their clients, as well as the clients themselves. This paper has described a systems orientation to the understanding of family problems as it can apply to aging families. By recognizing that the aged are members of a family system, social workers have an opportunity for meaningful intervention in the system to relieve many of the stresses that accompany the normal vicissitudes of aging.

REFERENCES

1. Streib, Gordon, "Family Patterns in Retirement" *Journal of Social Issues* 14:2, 1958, 46-60; Schorr, Alvin, *Filial Responsibility in the Modern American Family*, Washington, D.C.: Social Security Administration, 1960.
2. Bengtson, Vern L. and Treas, Judith, "The Changing Family Context of Mental Health and Aging" in Birren and Sloane, eds., *Handbook of Mental Health and Aging*, Englewood Cliffs, New Jersey: Prentice-Hall, Inc. 1980, 400.
3. Troll, Lillian E., Miller, S.J., and Atchley, R.C., *Families in Later Life*, Belmont, California: Wadsworth Publishing Co., Inc., 1979.
4. Ackerman, Nathan A., *The Psychodynamics of Family Life*, New York: Basic Books, 1958.
5. Troll, Miller, and Atchley, *op.cit.*
6. Simos, Bertha G., "Adult Children and Their Aging Parents" *Social Work* 18:3, 1973, 78-85.
7. Monk, Abraham, "Family Supports in Old Age" *Social Work* 24:6, 1979, 533-539.
8. *Natural Supports Program List of Publications* September 1981, Community Service Society, 105 East 22nd Street, New York, New York 10010.
   Silverstone, Barbara, and Hyman, Helen K. *You and Your Aging Parent*, New York: Pantheon Books, 1982.

Presentations at the Thirty-Third Annual Meeting of The Gerontological Society of America, San Diego, California, November, 1980: Horowitz, Amy and Shindelman, Lois, *The Impact of Caregiving for an Elderly Relative*; Kirschner, Charlotte, *The Role of Skilled Family Counselling in Maintaining the Elderly at Home*; Mellor, Joanna and Getzel, George, *Stress and Service Needs of Those Who Care for the Aged*; Zweibel, N.R. *The Impact of Parent-Caring on the Middle-Aged Child.*

9. O'Connell, P., "Family Developmental Tasks" *Smith College Studies in Social Work* 42:6, June, 1972, 203-210.

10. Erikson, Erik H., "Identity and the Life Cycle" *Psychological Issues* 1:1, 1959, New York: International Universities Press.

11. Presentations at the Thirty-Fourth Annual Meeting of The Gerontological Society of America, Toronto, Canada, November, 1981: Brody, Elaine M., Johnsen, P.T., and Fulcomer, M.C. What Should Adult Children Do for Elderly Parents: Expectations of Three Generations of Women; Danis, B. and Silverstone, Barbara, Sources of Conflict for Middle-Aged Daughters and Older Wives in Caregiving Situations; Horowitz, Amy, Sons and Daughters as Caregivers to Older Parents: Differences in Role Performance and Consequences.

12. Boszormenyi-Nagy, I., and Spark, G. *Invisible Loyalties*, New York: Harper and Row, 1973.

13. Silverstone, Barbara, and Hyman, Helen K. *You and Your Aging Parent*, New York: Pantheon Books, 1982.

14. Report to the Congress by the Comptroller General of the United States, Washington, D.C.: December 30, 1977.

15. *Aging Parents: Whose Responsibility?* (A Workshop Model for Family Life Education) Family Service Association of America, 44 East 23rd Street, New York, New York 10010; *As Parents Grow Older: A Manual for Program Replication*, Institute of Gerontology, The University of Michigan, Ann Arbor, Michigan 48109; *Developing a Training Program for Families of the Mentally Impaired Aged*, Isabella Geriatric Center, 515 Audubon Avenue, New York, New York 10040; *Support Groups for Caregivers of the Aged: A Training Manual for Facilitators*, Community Service Society, 105 East 22nd Street, New York, New York, 10010; *The Aging Parent: A Guide for Program Planners*, The American Jewish Committee, 165 East 56th Street, New York, New York 10022.

16. Silverstone and Hyman, *op. cit.*

17. Headley, L., *Adults and Their Parents in Family Therapy*, New York: Plenum Press, 1977; Herr, J.J. and Weakland, J.H., *Counselling Elders and Their Families*, New York: Springer Publishing Co., 1979; Kirschner, Charlotte, "The Aging Family in Crisis; A Problem in Living" *Social Casework* 60:4, April, 1979, 209-216.

18. Napier, A.Y., with Whitaker, C.A., *The Family Crucible*, New York: Harper and Row, 1978.

19. Minuchin, Salvador, *Families and Family Therapy*, Boston: Harvard University Press, 1974.

20. Blenkner, Margaret, "Social Work and Family Relationships in Later Life with Some Thoughts on Filial Maturity" *Social Structure and the Family*, Shanas, Elaine and Streib, Gordon, eds., Englewood Cliffs, New Jersey: Prentice Hall, 1965.

21. Minuchin, Salvador, *op. cit.*

22. Kirschner, Charlotte, "The Aging Family in Crisis: A Problem in Living" *Social Casework* 60:4, April, 1979, 209-216.

23. Schulman, Gerda L., "Teaching Family Therapy to Social Work Students" *Social Casework* 57:7, July 1976, 448-457.

24. Comfort, Alex, *Practice of Geriatric Psychiatry*, New York: Elsevier Press, 1980, 71.

25. Kirschner, Charlotte, *op. cit.*

26. Krill, Donald, "Family Interviewing as an Intake Diagnostic Method," *Social Work* 13:4, April, 1968, 56-63.

27. Schulman, Gerda L., *op. cit.*

28. Neugarten, Bernice L., *Middle Age and Aging*, Chicago: University of Chicago Press, 1968.
29. Getzel, George S., "Helping Elderly Couples in Crisis," *Social Casework*, 63:9 Nov. 1982, 515-521.
30. Getzel, George S., *op. cit.*
31. Shanas, Elaine, *The Health of Older People: A Social Survey* Cambridge, Massachusetts: Harvard University Press, 1962.

Chapter V

Developments in Protective Services: A Challenge for Social Workers

Elizabeth Zborowsky

Protective services for older people emerged as a social welfare issue in the United States in the mid 1950's, quickly grew into a minor social movement during the 1960's, and then vanished from social work practice literature after the early 1970's. The sudden loss of interest in the further development of protective practice defies an easy explanation. The number of older people vulnerable to abuse, neglect, and exploitation has continued to grow along with the general increase in the U.S. population aged 65 and older. It is estimated that between 10 to 15 percent, or 3 to 4 million, elderly persons are in need of protective services.[1] It also appears that the incidence of elder abuse may be much higher than previously suspected.[2]

Furthermore, the effectiveness of the protective casework model in use since the 1960's remains questionable.[3] Yet, there are few reports of efforts to refine and reevaluate this model or to apply some of the newer social work practice models to the problems of abuse, neglect, and exploitation of older people.

Although these are all logical arguments for the further development of protective practice, this seems unlikely to occur until such time when current practice begins to be questioned. Therefore, the aim here is to rekindle social workers' curiosity about protective practice by analyzing the development of protective services for older people and some of the unresolved issues.

CASE ILLUSTRATIONS

Analyses usually begin with definitions to establish a common understanding of the subject matter. However, protective services for older people, like most other human services, has no one generally accepted definition. Consequently, the following case illustrations are used instead of definitions to describe the kinds of situations involving protective services for older people. These case situations, cited in the reports of three of the protective research and demonstration projects, reflect the problems of self or other inflicted abuse, neglect, and exploitation of older people.

> Mrs. B. frequently calls old age assistance worker complaining that son beats her with a cane. Story substantiated by physician and by neighbors. Client up in wheelchair at times but mainly bedfast. Has glaucoma and arteriosclerosis. . . Police frequently called and son denies mistreatment. Mrs. B. pleads to go to a nursing home and then will deny in front of son. Son resists all attempts to place mother. Son is married and living with wife in Mrs. B.'s home. Caseworker has seen son's wife intoxicated. Son is a heavy drinker and does odd jobs—no steady employment. . .[4]

A woman living alone refused to have a doctor, although a leg infection had become so critical that without immediate medical care she would likely die. Her house was in complete disorder and her several cats were obviously starving. She was sure that the patent medicine she was taking would make her well.[5]

Mr. L., aged 67, was referred by the Public Health district nurse because of potential exploitation. The protective service staff found him living in a most primitive way, sleeping in a hall closet and surviving on coffee, doughnuts, and wine. He had recently qualified for Social Security benefits and soon was to receive a sizeable lump sum. He suffered from severe memory loss, and it was obvious to the workers that he was not competent to manage either his funds or personal life and that his landlord and others were using his money for their own benefit.[6]

EARLY LEGAL AND SOCIAL SERVICE PERSPECTIVES

Protective services for older people involve legal and social issues. During the first half of the twentieth century the main forms of protective services for adults were the states' legal procedures for commitment to a state mental hospital or for the appointment of a guardian. However, the limitations of these legal interventions became more apparent in the mid 1950's when more older people were eligible to receive monthly government benefit checks. The Social Security Administration, the Veterans Administration, and the American Public Welfare Association were confronted with an increased number of recipients of retirement and old age assistance benefits who evidenced serious difficulties in handling their checks. Most of these older people did not require psychiatric hospitalization. At the same time it was usually not possible for them to pay the fees for a court appointed guardian to help them manage their affairs in the community. The three agencies eventually dealt with the problem by establishing procedures for making a relative or other interested person the "representative payee" for the older person's check. Despite various safeguards, the representative payee procedure has been used to exploit some older people.[7] It also raises many unresolved constitutional issues.[8]

The problems of these marginally competent older people in managing their affairs also became more visible to the general public, particularly to bankers, lawyers, physicians, and social welfare agencies. The horrendous environmental conditions under which some of them lived and their frequent resistance to the regular community services led to widespread pressure for the development of specialized protective social services.

PROTECTIVE SOCIAL WORK PRACTICE

During the 1960's the development of protective services for older people was approached with a missionary-like zeal that was later described as having some of the characteristics of a minor social movement.[9] In 1963 The National Council on the Aging published the first study of the social and legal implications of protective services.[10] It served as a basic resource for a series of interdisciplinary—law, health care, and social welfare—conferences held across the country. The purposes of these seminars, described in some of the published proceedings, were to define protective services, to develop practical guidelines for community based protective service programs, and to stimulate communities to develop their own programs.[11]

In addition seven major protective service research and demon-

stration projects were conducted in different parts of the country.
The projects were under the auspices of various types of agencies as
follows: The Benjamin Rose Institute in Cleveland;[12] the coordinated agencies service model in Chicago;[13] The National Council
on the Aging studies at the Sheltering Arms in Houston, the Protective Service Agency in San Diego, and the Public Welfare Department in Philadelphia;[14] the Administration on Aging study of the
Protective Service Agency in San Diego;[15] and the Community Service Administration National Protective Service Project for Older
Adults at the Public Welfare Departments of Washington, D.C. and
the three rural Colorado counties of Morgan, Weld, and Logan.[16]

These protective service research and demonstration projects provided descriptive information about their respective clients and services. Some also used the data to develop problem and social work
intervention typologies. Ferguson[17] compiled a table which sum-
marized some of the descriptive data about the protective clients
served by each of the projects. Although the data were not strictly
comparable, they did suggest that the clients tended to be aged 75 or
older, females, white, and currently not married. Furthermore, they
usually lived alone in a private house or apartment and were not
totally destitute by 1960's income standards.

The Benjamin Rose Institute Study

In addition to collecting descriptive data The Benjamin Rose Institute project, Protective Services for Older People,[18] used an
experimental research design to test the effectiveness of the demonstration service. Older persons referred to the project between June
1964 and June 1965 were randomly assigned to receive the
demonstration protective service (N = 76 in the experimental
group) or the usual community services (N = 88 in the control
group). Structured research interviews were conducted at regular
intervals with all 164 participants and their respective collaterals. It
was hypothesized that the experimental service group would have
higher contentment scores and survival rates than the control group.
Such a finding would indicate that the Institute's specialized protective services were more effective than the usual community services for this particular group of older people.

The older person in need of protective services was defined as
follows:

A noninstitutionalized person 60 years of age or older living in the community whose behavior indicates that he is mentally incapable of adequately caring for himself and his interests without serious consequences to himself or others and has no relative or other private individual able and willing to assume the kind and degree of support and supervision required to control the situation.[19]

The Institute's protective service model consisted of social casework as the core service and seven ancillary services—financial, medical, home aide, social service assistant, placement, fiduciary, and guardianship services and legal and psychiatric consultation. All of these services were of "best quality possible" and provided by the Institute "in the maximum quantity." Clients' other needs, for example housing, were met through the use of other community resources.[20]

Social casework practice, the core service in the model, was based on a psychoanalytic orientation which emphasized the worker's use of relationship and psychodynamic understanding of clients' personalities. The service goals were psychotherapeutic in terms of helping clients with severe mental impairment to make a better functional adaptation to their limitations and surroundings. However, the goals were also sociotherapeutic in that the ancillary services were used to protect clients from abuse, neglect, or exploitation and to ameliorate their frequently untenable living conditions.[21]

MSW caseworkers carried primary responsibility for making the diagnostic assessment and treatment plan, serving the client directly, managing/directing the ancillary services and staff, and coordinating the use of other community resources. The dictum to the caseworker was, "Do or get others to do, all that was necessary to meet the demands of the situation, whatever the magnitude of the client's social and personal pathology."[22]

Contrary to the predicted outcome, the study findings showed that the Institute's specialized protective services were not more effective than the usual community control services. The experimental service group failed to achieve significantly higher contentment scores or survival rates. In fact the intensive experimental services appeared to increase the chance of death which was associated with a higher rate of institutionalization, used as a protective intervention.[23]

These unexpected findings aroused considerable controversy

among social work practitioners and research methodologists.[24] Unfortunately, Margaret Blenkner's sudden death in 1973 precluded further clarification of some of the issues. The Institute has recently completed a reanalysis of the original project data, using more recently developed statistical procedures. Their forthcoming report may provide some new insights on the findings.

Hiatus in the Development of Protective Practice

The Institute's study was the first of the protective service research and demonstration projects. Its service model[25] with some variations in the component services and/or the roles of the ancillary staff became the basis for most of the protective practice described in the literature. However, after the publication of the final reports of the research and demonstration projects in the early 1970's, the discussion of protective practice with older people in essence vanished from the professional literature.

One exception was an article by Hobbs (1976) on the development of short-term individual and group service protective practice at the San Diego County Welfare Department. In order to design innovative protective services for older people Hobbs urged that the usual approach of starting with the definition of the component services be put aside. Instead, she recommended defining the objective to be achieved by the service first, the process essential for achievement of the objective next, and the component services necessary to implement the program last.[26] Such an approach would encourage the evaluation of the effectiveness of the protective services in achieving the objectives. However, it still could constrain innovative thinking about protective practice, if the objectives were defined in terms of existing services.

Another exception was a monograph by Ferguson (1978) which dealt with adult protective service policy and program issues and recommendations. Of particular interest for the protective service practitioner was her framework for case decision making. A flow chart identified thirteen decisions a protective service worker with older people would be likely to make. For each decision Ferguson outlined the types and standards of evidence needed to make the decision and some alternative responses to clients and the respective consequences.[27] It is not a panacea for working with resistive clients in need of protective services. However, it does provide a tool for the worker to use in sorting out a client's situation, defining relation-

ships among various community resources, clarifying agency policy, and deciding on the most appropriate course of action.

RECENT LEGAL PERSPECTIVES

Despite the waning interest in the further development of protective social work practice over the past decade, protective services
for older people has remained a viable legal and social welfare
issue. Legally, there has been a growing concern about the rights of
older people in need of protective services; for example their right
to refuse service, the failure of existing guardianship laws to meet
the needs of marginally competent adults, and the tendency of the
courts to handle guardianship proceedings in a very perfunctory
manner. The last issue has been especially critical for older people,
since guardianship is often the prelude to placement in a nursing
home against their wishes followed by their loss of hope and then
death.

To address some of these problems Regan and Springer[28]
prepared a working paper for the U.S. Congress. In it they proposed
model statutes for state legislators to consider. These included: an
adult protective services act; guardianship, conservatorship of property, and power of attorney legislation; a public guardian act; and
amendments to state civil commitment laws. A 1980 survey showed
that 25 states had adopted some type of adult protective services
law, another 14 had legislation pending, and 4 states were in the
process of drafting legislation. Of the 25 states with adult protective
service laws, 16 of these laws were adopted between the years of
1975 and 1980.[29]

ELDER ABUSE

The most recent development in adult protective services has
been the concern about elder abuse as a national social problem. The
public's increasing awareness of the problem is reflected in the
reports of at least two Congressional hearings.[30] The results of the
following exploratory, epidemiological, research surveys of professionals with first hand knowledge of the problem of elder abuse have
also been published. These surveys were conducted in the Greater
Washington, D.C. S.M.S.A. located in Maryland;[31] in Michigan;[32]

in Cleveland at the Chronic Illness Center;[33] in Massachusetts[34] and in Southern Maine-Northern New Hampshire.[35] Since all of these surveys were limited to convenience samples of professionals in the human services, the results have to be considered highly speculative. Nevertheless, they do suggest some tentative patterns in the problem of elder abuse for further study. White females, aged 80 and older, with a major physical or mental disability that prevented them from meeting their own daily needs seemed to be at the greatest risk for abuse. They tended to live with others and in the same household as their abusers. The abusers were most often adult children; less than 20 percent of the reported abuse was inflicted by a nonrelative. The surveys differed on whether physical or verbal/emotional abuse occurred more frequently, and no single causal explanation for the abuse predominated.

The elder abuse survey findings also suggested that some type of professional intervention took place in most of the situations despite initial resistances and barriers to service. However the professionals varied considerably in their judgments about their success in resolving the elder abuse problem. Of particular interest in light of the earlier findings of Blenkner et al.[36] was the frequency with which the elder abuse problem was addressed by removing the elderly victims from their homes.[37] Like the protective service research and demonstration projects of the 1960's, the elder abuse surveys of the 1980's continue to point out the need for new, more effective approaches to protective practice.

ISSUES AND QUESTIONS

The foregoing literature review suggests several issues whose exploration might facilitate the further development of protective services for older people. The article by Hobbs[38] raises a key issue with regard to the past emphasis on beginning with the definition of the component services required for the delivery of protective services. Although it may be more comfortable for social workers to start with what is most familiar (social services) this is problematic for two reasons. Firstly it tends to limit innovation since the component service definitions reflect existing services. Secondly, it bases the design of protective services more on what professionals know how to do than on the changing needs of older people vulnerable to abuse, neglect, and exploitation. New protective service programs which start with defining the component services they will provide seem to result not in innovative approaches but in more of the same services.

A second issue concerns the identification of the social problem which protective services are expected to change. Is the "older person in need of protective services" the social problem as suggested by Bloom and Nielsen?[39] Is it the acts, whether self or other inflicted, of abuse, neglect, and exploitation of older people? How the problem gets defined is significant for protective practice because it determines who is included and excluded from the target population. It also influences the choice of social theories used to explain the problem and to prescribe social work interventions.

For example, in the protective service literature, the problem has usually been implicitly identified as the individual older person unable to manage his/her own affairs. Consequently, protective practice has for the most part been limited to a traditional casework approach. However, if the problem were identified as the abuse, neglect, and exploitation of older people, would this encourage the testing of family unit treatment models in situations of elder abuse by others? Would the ecological model[40] be especially well suited to dealing with the often conflicting goals of protective services—to protect the older person from abuse, neglect, or exploitation; to uphold his civil rights; and to preserve the general welfare of society? The ecological model is directed toward improving the transactions between people and environments in order to enhance the adaptive capacities and improve environments for all who function within them.

A separate but related issue, the definition of the problem, is a critical link to developing innovative approaches to protective services for older people. If the problem is defined in terms of its most desirable outcome, disregarding the issues of barriers or feasibilities, it encourages more creative thinking about possible ways to achieve this outcome.[41] These ideal services can later be modified to meet the constraints of the real world. However, beginning with the most desirable outcome for the problem can provide a way to move beyond the currently existing ideas about protective practice.

This also raises the interesting question of what is the most desirable outcome of protective services? Is it to protect or shield older people from the effects of abuse, neglect, or exploitation? Is it to stop or prevent the abuse, neglect, or exploitation of older people? The former tends to justify interventions involving the institutionalization of vulnerable older people. The latter requires a much broader focus than the older person in need of protective services. A prerequisite for the latter is the further study of abuse, neglect, and exploitation, barely begun by the recent exploratory elder abuse surveys.

The fourth and final protective services issues to be considered here are the new protective service laws in many states. Those laws, patterned after the Regan and Springer model statutes, provide a legal basis for designated social workers to assess the need for and deliver protective services, even though the older person or a caretaker resists such intervention. However, protective service workers must be knowledgeable about the laws in their respective states and conduct their practice within the provisions of these laws. For example, some of the laws include legal definitions for abstract concepts such as "hazardous living conditions," "incapacitated person," "protective placement," and even "protective services." They also establish legal guidelines and criteria for the delivery of protective services. These include: geriatric evaluations; voluntary protective services; involuntary court ordered protective services, emergency services, and placement services; court hearing and petition procedures; mandatory reporting of suspected abuse, neglect, or exploitation of adults; and the older person's right to appeal court ordered protective services or placement.[42]

The aim of these laws is to assure the well-being of older people and at the same time to protect their civil rights. These laws integrate the legal and social service aspects of protective services for older people in new ways. However, the laws are based on existing protective service social work practice, originally developed in the 1960's. Therefore, it seems doubtful that the laws themselves will lead to innovative protective practice.

The search for more effective protective social services requires a continuous, helical process of rethinking practice issues and questions, implementing services designed to achieve the most desirable outcome, evaluating the effectiveness of the services in producing the desired outcome, and then rethinking the issues, modifying the services, and reevaluating ad infinitum. The further development of protective social work practice does not promise to be an easy task, but effective protective services are vital to the well-being of older people vulnerable to abuse, neglect, or exploitation.

REFERENCES

1. Regan, J.J. & Springer, G. *Protective Services for the Elderly A Working Paper* (U.S. Congress, Senate, Special Committee on Aging). Washington, D.C.: Government Printing Office, 1977.
2. U.S. Congress, Senate, Special Committee on Aging (96th Congress, 1st session). *Elder Abuse: the Hidden Problem.* Washington, D.C.: U.S. Government Printing Office, 1979.
   U.S. Congress, Senate, Special Committee on Aging, & House, Select Committee on Aging (96th Congress, 2nd session). *Elder Abuse.* Washington, D.C., 1980.
3. Blenkner, M., Bloom, M., & Nielson, M. A research and demonstration project of protective services. *Social Casework.* 1971, *52*, 483-499.
   Blenkner, M., Bloom, M., Nielson, M., & Weber, R. *Final report. Protective Services for Older People Findings from the Benjamin Rose Institute Study* (Pt. 1). Cleveland: Benjamin Rose Institute, 1974.
4. Ibid., p. 23.
5. Hall, G.H., & Mathiasen, G. (Eds.) *Guide to development of protective services for older people.* Foreword by Jack Ossofsky. Springfield, Illinois: Charles C Thomas, 1973.
6. U.S. Dept. of Health, Education and Welfare, Community Services Act. 1971, p.69.
7. Hall, G.H. Protective services for adults. *Encyclopedia of Social Work* (Vol. 2, 16th issue). New York: National Association of Social Workers, 1971.
8. Regan, J.J. & Springer, G. Op. cit.
9. Blenkner, M. *Prevention or Protection? Aspects of social welfare service for the mentally impaired aged.* Paper presented at the 1st Workshop on Comprehensive Services for the Geriatric Mental Patient, 30 Nov.-Dec.1st 1967. (Available from Librarian, The Benjamin Rose Institute, 636, Rose Bldg., Cleveland, Ohio 44115.)
10. Lehmann, V., & Mathiasen, G., *Guardianship and protective services for older people.* New York: National Council on Aging, 1963.
11. Eckstein, R., & Lindey, E. (Eds.) *Seminar on protective services for older people. Proceedings of a seminar held at Arden House, Harriman, New York. March 10-15, 1963.* New York: National Council on the Aging, 1964.
    Hall, G.H., & Mathiasen, G. (Eds.) *Overcoming Barriers to protective services for the aged.* New York: National Council on the Aging, 1968.
    Hughes, M.R. (Ed.) *Protective services for older adults. Workshop proceedings of a conference.* Portland, Oregon: Friendly House, 1968.
    Lindey, E. (Ed.) *A Crucial issue in social work practice. Protective services for older people.* New York: National Council on the Aging, 1966.
    Lynes, J.K. *The evaluation of protective services for older people.* San Diego: Community Welfare Council of San Diego, 1970.
12. Blenkner, M., Bloom, M., & Nielson, M. Op. cit.
    Blenkner, M., Bloom, M., Nielson, M., & Weber, R. Op. cit.
    Wasser, E. Protective practice in serving the mentally impaired aged. *Social Casework*, 1971, *52*, 510-522.
    Wasser, E. *Protective casework practice with older people: An explication of the service component in the Benjamin Rose Institute study* (Pt. 2). Cleveland: Benjamin Rose Institute, 1974.
13. Council for Community Services in Metropolitan Chicago. *Protective services for the aged* (Publication No. 7401). Chicago: Zborowsky, 1973.
    Council for Community Services in Metropolitan Chicago. *Final Report of services to impaired aged pilot program* (Publication No. 7503). Chicago: Zborowsky, 1975.
14. Hall, G.H. & Mathiasen, G. (eds.) 1973 Op. cit.
15. Horowitz, G., & Estes, C. *Protective services for the aged* (U.S. Dept. of Health,

Education and Welfare, Adminstration on Aging). Washington, D.C.   U.S. Government Printing Office, 1971.
16. U.S. Community Services Act, 1971 Op.cit.
17. Ferguson, E.J. *Protecting the Vulnerable Adult* Ann Arbor, Michigan: University of Michigan-Wayne State University, Institute of Gerontology, 1978.
18. Blenkner et al., 1971 Op.cit.
    Blenkner et al., 1974 Op.cit.
    Wasser, E. 1971 Op.cit.
    Wasser, E. 1974 Op. cit.
19. Weber, R. Definition of an older person in need of protective service used in the B.R.I. study (Appendix A). In M. Blenkner, M. Bloom, M. Nielson, & R. Weber, *Final Report. Protective services for older people findings from the Benjamin Rose Institute study* (Pt. 1 p.205). Cleveland: Benjamin Rose Institute, 1974.
20. Blenkner et al., 1971 Op.cit.
    Blenkner et al., 1974 Op.cit.
21. Wasser, 1971 Op.cit.
    Wasser, 1974 Op.cit.
22. Ibid. p.12
23. Blenkner et al., 1971 Op. cit.
    Blenkner et al., 1974 Op. cit.
24. Berger, R.M., & Piliavin, I. The effect of casework: A research note. *Social Work,* 1976, *21*, 205-208.
    Berger, R.M., & Piliavin, I. A rejoinder by Berger and Piliavin. *Social Work,* 1976, *21*, 349;396-397.
    Fischer, J. Is casework effective? A review. *Social Work,* 1973, *18*, 5-20.
    Fischer, J., & Hudson, W.W. An effect of casework? Back to the Drawing board. *Social Work,* 1976, *21*, 347-349.
    Wagner, D., & Osmalov, M.J. *The impact of social casework on the elderly: A reappraisal of the controversy surrounding the Benjamin Rose Institute's protective services study.* Unpublished manuscript, 1978. (Available from the librarian, The Benjamin Rose Institute, 636, Rose Bldg., Cleveland, Ohio 44115).
25. Wasser, E. 1971 Op. cit.
    Wasser, E. 1974 Op. cit.
26. Hobbs, L. Adult protective services: A new program approach. *Public Welfare,* 1976, *34*, 28-37.
27. Ferguson, E.J., 1978 Op. cit.
28. Regan, J.J. & Springer, G., 1977 Op. cit.
29. U.S. Congress, 1980 Op. cit.
30. Ibid.
    U.S. Congress, 1979 Op. cit.
31. Block, M.R., & Sinnott, J.D. Methodology and Results. In M.R. Block & J.D. Sinnott (Eds), *Battered Elder Syndrome: An exploratory study.* College Park, Maryland: University of Maryland, Center on Aging, 1979. pp.67-84.
32. Hickey, T., & Douglass, R.L. Neglect and Abuse of older family members: Professionals' perspectives and case experiences. *Gerontologist,* 1981, *21*, pp.171-176.
33. Lau, E.E., & Kosberg, J.I. Abuse of the elderly by informal care providers. *Aging,* 1979 (Nos. 299-300), 10-15.
34. Legal Research and Services for the elderly. Elder Abuse in Massachusetts: A survey of professionals and paraprofessionals. In U.S. Congress, House, Select Committee on Aging, *Elder Abuse the hidden problem* (96th Congress, 1st session). Washington, D.C.; U.S. Government Printing Office, 1979.
35. McLaughlin, J.S., Nickell, J.P., & Gill, L. An epidemiological investigation of elderly abuse in Southern Maine and New Hampshire, 1979-80. In U.S. Congress, Senate, Special committee on Aging & House, Select committee on Aging, *Elder Abuse* (96th Congress, 2nd. session). Washington, D.C.: Government Printing Office, 1980.

36. Blenkner, M. et al., 1971 Op.cit.
Blenkner, M. et al., 1974 Op.Cit.
37. Lau, E.E. & Kosberg, J.I. Op. cit.
Legal Research and Services for the Elderly. 1979. Op.cit.
38. Hobbs, L. 1976 Op.cit.
39. Bloom, M., & Nielson, M. The older person in need of protective services. *Social Casework*, 1971, *52*,500-509.
Bloom, M., & Nielson, M. The protective as a social problem. In M. Blenkner, M. Bloom, M. Nielson, & R. Weber, *Final Report. Protective services for older people findings from the Benjamin Rose Institute study* (Pt. 1). Cleveland: Benjamin Rose Institute, 1974.
40. Germain, Carol B. (Ed.) *Social Work Practice: People and environments an ecological perspective.* New York: Columbia University Press, 1979.
41. Blum, Arthur *Delivery systems and service delivery.* Course 694 at Case Western Reserve University, School of Applied Social Sciences, Cleveland. Spring 1981.
42. Regan, J.J. & Springer, G., 1977 Op. cit.

Chapter VI

Outreach to the Elderly: Community Based Services

Cynthia Stuen

INTRODUCTION

Community outreach is a component of many community based social service agencies. Frequently mandated by legislation, outreach seeks to locate and link the population in need with the services available. Exploration of the various issues and methods of outreach relative to community based services for the elderly is the objective of this chapter. Specific attention will be given to the issue of reaching minority older persons.

Structural Forms of Service Delivery

The present structure of the continuum of services available to the elderly ranges from community, neighborhood based services to institutional care, including care for the terminally ill, frequently referred to as hospice. Tobin identifies three structures which incorporate the range of health and social services now available.[1]

First, community based organizations focus on the well elderly working to prevent premature or unnecessary institutionalization. Typical services in this category are information, referral, casework, home health, transportation/escort, volunteer, friendly visiting, telephone reassurance and meals on wheels. The second structure encompasses long term care institutions. These facilities are congregate settings providing 24 hour custodial and some rehabilitative care and are generally referred to as skilled nursing and intermediate care facilities. Domiciliary care facilities provide a bed and board service and are part of this structure. It is proposed by Tobin that these be small humane facilities in local communities linked to larger primary care facilities for back up. The third structure emerges out of the English hospice movement for the terminally ill. As deaths become more concentrated in the latter part of the life span with increasing dependence on institutional settings for death, this structure is likely to increase substantially in the years ahead. While terminal care is presently thought of as occurring in a separate facility, indications are that this too will become a service of in-home care at the neighborhood level.

This analysis brings one full circle to the need for a coordinated approach to care based in the community. A cadre of support services, needed by individuals and their families in a neighborhood setting is and must be a high priority for social planners. Recognition of minority groups within the community and their cultural differences in viewing services within a neighborhood is an important ingredient as services and outreach methods are planned. However, caution needs to be exercised in that there are no simple solutions to providing services for minority elderly. "Separate services" are not always an answer nor is an integrated approach, "one size fits all," as described by Taylor,[2] always an appropriate response. A discussion of this policy issue is not appropriate to this chapter but is mentioned only to highlight its importance for the planning phase of community based services.

Development of Community Based Organization

The Social Security Act, landmark legislation of 1935, characterized a nation's concern for its elderly. However, it has only been in the last fifteen years that service programs have emerged for the elderly. Passage of the Social Security Amendments of Title XVIII (Medicare) and Title XIX (Medicaid) in 1965 gave further recognition to the plight of elderly, and other indigent age groups, in obtaining affordable health care. The greatest growth occurred in the institutional settings for health services delivery as nursing homes proliferated, particularly in the private profit making sector. The resulting escalation in spending for Medicare and Medicaid prompted increased concern for alternatives to the institutional model and emergence in the 1970's of concerns for home care and other community based service alternatives.

The Older Americans Act (1965) marked the beginning of a new era. The federal government moved beyond income supplementation to funding services with eligibility being determined purely on the basis of age (60), not need. The Older Americans Act (OAA) covers a wide range of activities and many sections of the act mandated outreach services. The OAA funded services are divided into two classifications. Part one are the formal services delivered in-home including home delivered meals, homemaker/chore, home repair, friendly visiting, and telephone reassurance. These are usually provided on a one-to-one basis. Part two are out-of-home services or congregate site services including senior centers, nutrition programs, and group transportation services. Title XX of the Social Security Act funds some services for elderly which enhance or replicate the OAA funded ones.

Jacqueline Johnson Jackson's work on minorities and aging provides an important understanding of the difficulty that aged minorities, who are poor and poorly educated, tend to have in finding their way through the maze of federally funded programs. Her work also poignantly reminds practitioners not only of the heterogeneity of the elderly but the heterogeneity within each minority group. A case in point is a statement by a representative of the National Puerto Rican Forum who stated that New York City's Hispanic community originates from eighteen different countries, each demanding a different service and outreach response. From a planning perspective Johnson recommends planning for groups within minority populations.[3]

In addition to the formal service network, older adults rely on the family network as a major provider of supports at the time when their dependencies increase. Therefore inclusion of the family/nonfamily support network in outreach strategies can be most appropriate. Eugene Litwak believes that in all areas of life there will be aspects of a given task for which the family will be superior to the formal organizations, and other aspects for which the opposite will hold true.[4]

Recently, the informal service network has been gaining recognition for its value to the formal service organizations. While no official funding source supports these projects, demonstration grants have shown the value of programs for caregivers of the elderly. The Community Service Society of New York has been a leader in this area through its Natural Supports Program.[5] Volunteer groups, religious groups, civic and service organizations have all joined in fostering the informal networks of older persons and/or their "informal supports."

Definition and Purpose of Outreach

Outreach is an effort to link people in need to appropriate community resources. Outreach takes the services of information and referral out of an agency or center into the community. A variety of outreach strategies is discussed later in this chapter.

There are two perspectives from which to approach outreach. One is on behalf of a singular program with the goal of locating, informing and persuading persons to become participants in that program. The program seeks to assure community awareness and to identify and recruit the target population for which the service is designed. If outreach is successful, appropriate utilization of the resource is accomplished. Hence accountability for the funding source is insured and contractual obligations to service the target population are fulfilled. Outreach from a community nutrition site is one such example.

The other perspective, while it may be from the vantage point of a single agency's outreach program, is a more generalist approach. A Title IIIb funded counseling service of the OAA illustrates this category whose goal is to identify persons in need and link them to available community resources. This perspective operates on the well documented assumption that people are often unaware of services that exist in the community. Added to this are psychosocial factors; fear of asking for help, denial of a problem, and the struggle to avoid "welfare." Agencies without an outreach component place the burden on the client to initiate service requests. The National Council on Aging demonstration, Project FIND, documented the necessity to proactively link the elderly with resources already in existence but unknown to the older person.[6]

Initial Phases of Outreach

Outreach includes determining needs, seeking funding and serving isolated elderly. This is substantiated by Project OPTIMIZE of the Massachusetts Association of Older Americans, a program utilizing older adults for outreach. Involvement of the community, particularly the elderly, in the process of a community needs assessment and planning process is imperative. It is important to obtain the views of the potential constituency and to learn their perception of needs and attitudes toward various services. Completion of the planning process before outreach begins, can make a critical difference in the acceptance of any new service. It also begins the process of outreach at the earliest moment of service conceptualization by allowing community input and hence "ownership" of the new service. As the need assessment and planning phases are in progress, potential recipients can be identified and a waiting list established for the day when the service is implemented. It also insures that the services to be offered are "acceptable" to the population in need.

At the point of program funding, it is necessary to clearly define the target population in terms of eligibility criteria such as age, geographical location, need, etc., and state the service or program limitations. These may need highlighting.

The recruitment and training of program staff and volunteers are steps in the implementation phase which should not be short-changed. The hiring of qualified staff and their training is the first phase of outreach. Each staff person brings to the program a network of personal and community contacts. Their effective reporting of new services will have a ripple effect in the community. Staff and volunteer awareness of their important role on and off the job should be discussed thoroughly in their orientation and training. It is of fundamental importance that outreach workers be aware of the entire array of services in the community and be competent in making accurate assessments of need and hence appropriate referrals and linkages. Ongoing training and information updating must be built into any agency's staff and volunteer development program, especially for those on the front line involved in outreach.

Outreach Strategies

There will never be a singular outreach strategy guaranteed to be effective in any given situation. Much will depend on the funding, staff and volunteer resources that a service or program has available to it as well as the extent of the appropriate outreach. Some programs are in such demand that outreach is not necessary for participant recruitment. If outreach is undertaken, it is important to be able to respond positively to requests for service. News in the community will travel very fast if there is a long waiting list and it will discourage future referrals. This situation is a "Catch 22" in that usually service expansion needs documentation but people get tired of calling when no help is offered. This can be addressed by careful explanation of service capability during outreach.

The common strategies for outreach are personal home visits, telephone contacts, personal letters and general printed materials. The focus can be individual enrollment or mass consumer enrollment. The individual services listed previously in the "in-home" category as well as congregate site activities will generally receive the best response from personal visits for recruitment.

A study investigating the relative success of different outreach methods with a group of low income elderly confirms the importance of a home visit for the success of enrolling participants in a senior center. The low income group is considered the most difficult group to reach but results showed the home visit received a 79% positive response, telephone contact received a 28% positive response, personal letter 11% and informational mail 2% positive responses. No response was documented from the control group who had been exposed to printed informational materials available in the community.[7]

When budgetary constraints do not allow for home visits, personalized letters and telephone contacts are suitable for outreach for noncrucial services. A follow up survey of the previously mentioned study reported that 59% of those receiving a personal letter and 78% a telephone call, remembered it and associated it appropriately when contacted one or two months later.

However, mass consumer enrollment is appropriate for broadly based community programs. Reduced fare transportation passes and other discount programs offered by merchants and the National Park Services utilize this strategy. To be effective, a mass consumer campaign must combine extensive publicity with easily accessible enrollment centers. Enrollment locations need to be at places such as shopping malls, health care facilities, senior centers, street fairs, and at any community event where the elderly are likely to congregate. While effective mass enrollment campaigns can recruit a large participant population, it will not locate the most needy, isolated older person. This population can only be reached through personalized approaches.

Outreach approaches to nonconsumers are also important for their community educational value and subsequent referral capacity. The traditional providers of social and health services are usually contacted, and, it is important not to limit outreach to just those agencies serving the elderly. Older persons are part of extended families and agencies serving the full life spectrum should be considered as targets for outreach. Persons in any of the helping professions should be oriented to the broad range of services for the entire age population whatever their work role. The office assistants in the private offices of physicians and therapists can be more important actors to orient to the services than the physicians or therapists themselves.

If a community does not have a general guide to services for all age groups, it may be necessary to list the services for the elderly in guides for other age groups until a comprehensive listing is recognized as a community need. Information about the service registered with special health related groups such as heart, lung, multiple sclerosis, ostomy clubs, etc. is important. Frequently these clubs have newsletters and welcome input on available resources.

Nontraditional outreach contacts can result in important linkages and expanded accessibility to community based services. The following illustrations of some nontraditional contacts are intended to encourage creativity in outreach. Elected officials and their staffs are often a first point of outreach by many persons in need. These officials have a vested interest in knowing community resources and are usually very receptive to information about new services. Public utilities have consumer divisions and may also publish a newsletter which is enclosed with monthly billing statements. Businesses in the community, particularly supermarkets, have community bulletin boards. Pharmacies and banks are frequented by the elderly and can be an important location for outreach brochures, posters or outposting of staff, for instance, especially on the first few days of the month when social security checks are being cashed. Religious institutions and civic associations can be utilized to help identify isolated persons within neighborhoods. Personal contact with their leadership is recommended as well as personal presentations to the appropriate groups.

Educational facilities such as public and private schools and their parent/teacher organizations are an often overlooked resource with which to share service information. Local libraries are becoming aware of their need to publicize resources and in New York City, a directory of community services is published by the public library system and available in each branch throughout the city. Newsletters of schools, colleges, and associations are always a "free" source of advertising.

Formation of a community advisory board or committee is another important strategy for outreach. Careful selection of board members can give the agency or program access to such media as newspapers, television, professional and business groups.

It is important to remember to check that one has utilized internal and informal relationships of the program's own staff and volunteers. One should not overlook any level of staff and never assume that staff will know everything that is going on by osmosis. A concerted effort to inform and update staff is essential.

Special Populations

Ethnic and cultural group factors have been shown to result in differential service utilization by the elderly. These factors should be considered in designing the services, especially the outreach.[8] Universal problems of aging interact with the behavior of the individual in the context of the culture and warrant attention in the service design and the outreach strategy. The cultural aspects are important in terms of how one approaches outreach so as not to violate or offend cultural traditions. In addition membership in a minority group is often associated with fewer opportunities than those experienced by the population as a whole and results in lower education and socioeconomic status and poorer health. When these factors are added to the problems concomitant with old age it is clear that ethnicity places older persons in "double jeopardy." Therefore, preferential consideration is essential in outreach.

The thrust of all service delivery systems, particularly as human service budgets shrink, is on efficiency. The 1978 amendments to the Older Americans Act emphasize "focal points of service delivery" which illustrates this point. The movement toward efficiency frequently entails centralization (focal points) where a lesser value is placed on grassroots, neighborhood based service delivery. A valid concern is, thus, whether "efficient, centrally accessible services" are utilized by the minority elderly. Too often, ethnicity is referred to as a descriptive variable in describing clients rather than being viewed as a critical ingredient in determining service approaches.[9]

A study of the utilization of community based services by minority older persons revealed that the strongest predictors of service to minorities were staffing patterns and location of program offices.[10] The study concluded that outreach will be most successful with minority groups when those staff conducting the outreach are of the same minority group, familiar with the neighborhood and the program is located within that neighborhood. Another predictor of agencies serving a proportionate share of minorities was that of door-to-door outreach or use of the media to publicize services. Agencies that provided staff training on the values and needs of minority older persons as well as agencies whose administrators believed in the importance of minority representation on their Board showed high usage by minority elderly in this study.

The implications of the research on serving minority elderly supports the need for ongoing outreach efforts, particularly door-to-door canvassing and telephone contacts. Bilingual staff and bilingual printed materials are also necessary for successful outreach. Location of the program within the minority neighborhood which recognizes the cultural differences of minority groups will maximize the opportunities for serving the minority elderly.

The rural elderly have been given a lesser status than the urban elderly in service development. Demographers began to track a reversal in the 1970's of the rural-to-urban population migration so that service delivery in rural areas may become a more important issue in the future. Not enough is known to say authoritatively that services to rural elderly should be "scaled down" versions of services to urban elderly. Rural outreach strategies also require further research. It is obvious that some of the resources taken for granted in an urban area can be major obstacles in a rural setting. Transportation, for instance, can be a critical obstacle to the accessing of services.

A major issue in addressing the rural elderly population is the diversity of this population. Another issue is the cost involved in providing the range of services for a diverse, sparsely populated group. A further challenge to service delivery and outreach is the independent spirit of rural America which downgrades acceptance of any service as "freeloading." This becomes a real challenge to workers to plan outreach strategies for services which must be portrayed in the least threatening way.[11]

The frail elderly, generally referring to the over 75 population who have physical or mental deficits, need special outreach attention. Personal contact is very essential to communicate with homebound, sensory impaired individuals. Sensitivity on the part of training of outreach workers to effectively communicate with the sight and hearing impaired as well as older adults with mental impairments is important. Materials in large type, tape recordings, public radio and television messages are techniques to be utilized. Outreach to the informal network for this vulnerable group is frequently the key to service utilization. Anyone surviving in the community with physical or mental impairments is likely to be reliant on an informal network, the members of which may be unaware of the formal service system. This caregiver network may be tapped through the workplace, religious organizations and any of the previously mentioned nonconsumer approaches.

Practical Considerations

Printed materials should be tailored for the intended readership, professional, lay or consumer. In addition to formal press releases, human interest stories highlighting a specific service will interest the lay reading audience more readily.

Public speaking to consumer and nonconsumer groups is important but care should be taken to utilize only the talents of "public speakers" among staff or volunteers. Preparation of visual aids such as posters, displays or slides to describe the agency's story can be accomplished without too much expense.

The burgeoning telecommunications field has far-reaching implications for outreach to older people. The existing television, radio and growing cable industry provide tremendous potential for public service information programming.

Two-way cable television with computer interface promises a future where an individual could access a program and obtain a comprehensive list of services available, select one, and then be contacted by that agency at home. One could project that door-to-door canvassing or personal visitation will someday be obsolete; however, this is not the case yet, nor have we faced some of the inherent problems of accessibility by those most in need. The issues of depersonalization, relations between professionals and clients, privacy, and confidentiality will remain.[12]

Barriers to Effective Outreach

A study of OAA Title VII Nutrition programs highlights some of the barriers to outreach and has implications for outreach in general.[13] The location of the meal site proved critical and a thorough needs assessment should document where the target population lives and identify the most accessible location before the site is selected. Location within a church or synagogue can result in interdenominational rivalry and may exclude a population in need. Outreach workers should be organized in pairs reflecting appropriate combinations of race, sex and age to facilitate recruitment The recruitment and training should emphasize the importance of positive relations in the community and how to help potential participants overcome their fear of going out to services or of receiving services in their home. A willingness to accept constituents on their terms of participation with maximum flexibility in eligibility is an important concept to instill within an agency.

In summary, barriers may be of a personal nature such as fear of participation; may be environmental, such as racial prejudice or programmatic, such as poor selection or inadequate transportation. Finally there is one additional principle to keep in mind. If, after utilizing all the appropriate strategies, success is not evident; ask "If people are not using this service, does the service itself need to be reexamined?" The line of questioning leads back to the needs assessment and planning phase and may suggest a new direction.

REFERENCES

1. Tobin, Sheldon, et al. *Effective Social Services for Older Americans.* Ann Arbor, Michigan: University of Michigan, 1976.
2. Taylor, S.P. Simple models of complexity: Programmatic considerations in providing service for minority elderly, In *Minority Aging; Policy issues for the 80's* E.P. Stanford, (Ed.). San Diego, California: The Campanile Press, 1981.
3. Jackson, J.J. *Minorities and Aging.* Belmont, California: Wadsworth Publishing Co., 1980.
    Jackson, J.J. Aged Negroes: Their cultural departures from statistical stereotypes and rural-urban differences, *Gerontologist* 10 (2), 1970: 140-145.
4. Litwak, E. Extended kin relations in an industrial democratic society. In Shanas, E. & Streib, G.F. (Eds.) *Social structure and the Family: Generational Relations.* New Jersey: Prentice Hall, Inc., 1965.
5. Zimmer, A.H. & Sainer, J.S. Strengthening the family as an informal support for their aged: Implications for social policy and planning. Paper presented at the 31st Annual Scientific meeting, Gerontological Society, Dallas, Texas. 1978.
6. National Council on Aging & the U.S. Office of Economic Opportunity. *The golden years: A Tarnished Myth* (Project Find). National Council on Aging, Washington, D.C., 1972.
7. Kushler, M.G. & W.S. Davidson, II, Alternative modes of outreach: An experimental comparison, *Gerontologist*, 18 (4), 1978: 355-362.
8. McCaslin, R. & Calvert, W.R. Social indicators in Black and White: Some ethnic considerations in delivery of service to the elderly, *Journal of Gerontology*, 30 (1), 1975: 60-66.
9. Jenkins, S. & Morrison, B. Ethnicity and service delivery, *American Journal of Orthopsychiatry*, 48 (1), 1978: 160-165.
10. Holmes, D. et al. The use of community based services in Long Term Care by older minority persons, *Gerontologist*, 19 (4), 1979: 389-397.

11. Coward, R.T. Planning community services for the rural elderly: Implications from research, *Gerontologist*, 19 (3), 1979: 275-282.
12. Black, K.D. & Bengston, V. Implications of telecommunications technology for old people, families and bureaucracies, In *Family, Bureaucracy and the Elderly*, E. Shanas & M.B. Sussman (Eds.), Durham, North Carolina: Duke University Press, 1977.
13. Schneider, L. Barriers to effective outreach in Title VII nutrition programs, *Gerontologist*, 19 (2), 1979: 163-168.

Section III

WITHIN THE AGED COHORT:
SPECIAL POPULATIONS AND NEEDS

Chapter VII

The Elderly Mentally Retarded: A Group in Need of Service

Marsha Mailick Seltzer
Gary B. Seltzer

Many gerontologists have explained that the elderly are not a homogeneous group,[1] but rather that they consist of a number of distinct subgroups, including the "young old" and the "old old"; the socially isolated elderly and those with a strong informal support network; institutionalized elderly and those who live in the community, etc. One subgroup that has received very little attention in the professional literature is the mentally retarded elderly. This group consists of mentally retarded persons who have survived to old age. They are distinct from the cognitively impaired elderly, who presumably had "normal" intelligence prior to growing older but who have some cognitive limitations due to Alzheimer's disease and other organic brain damage syndromes.

Like gerontologists, professionals in the field of mental retardation have argued that the mentally retarded are not a homogeneous group. Distinctions have been drawn among mildly, moderately, severely, and profoundly retarded persons; those who live in institutions and those who live in the community; those whose mental retardation was caused by a biochemical, physiological, or genetic disorder and those for whom the etiology of their mental retardation is unknown. Distinctions between retarded persons of various ages have been made, but these are primarily between retarded children and adults. Only a few articles have focused on elderly mentally retarded persons and attempted to examine this group for the purpose of identifying their special needs and characteristics.

The authors wish to gratefully acknowledge the contributions of Rose Ann Ariel, MSW and Alvin Rubin, MEd to this chapter.

The purpose of this chapter is to focus on the population of elderly mentally retarded persons and to identify social work practice issues and problems raised by this client population. Like the gerontology and mental retardation literatures, the social work literature has devoted very little attention to the elderly mentally retarded. For this reason, the present chapter will attempt to impart basic information about this client group as well as to identify the gaps in the research and practice literatures. Case examples will be presented to highlight key practice issues.

DEFINITION OF THE POPULATION

In order to develop a clear understanding of the special needs and characteristics of the group of individuals who are both elderly and mentally retarded, it is necessary first to attempt to develop a working definition of the parameters of this group. Most definitions of the elderly population in general have used age 65 as the minimum cut off point. In the mental retardation literature, "elderly" mentally retarded persons have been identified using considerably lower age cut off points, such as age 50,[2] age 55,[3] and age 60.[4] Tymchuk explains the use of younger ages to mark the onset of old age among the mentally retarded population on the basis of the apparent earlier onset of aging among retarded persons than among nonretarded persons.[5] However, he cautions that no empirical evidence exists supporting the hypothesis of their more rapid aging. Thus, the common use of demarcation points below age 65 for mentally retarded persons is somewhat arbitrary.

More clarity exists with respect to the definition of mental retardation, which is defined by the American Association on Mental Deficiency (AAMD) as:

Significantly subaverage general intellectual functioning existing concurrently with deficits in adaptive behavior, and manifested during the developmental period.[6]

Significantly subaverage general intellectual functioning refers to an IQ score at least two standard deviations below the population mean. The developmental period is defined as birth through 18 years. Adaptive behavior is defined as:

The effectiveness or degree with which an individual meets the standards of personal independence and social responsibility expected for age and cultural group.[6]

There are four levels of retardation: mild (IQ range approximately 55-69); moderate (IQ range approximately 40-54); severe (IQ range approximately 25-39); and profound (IQ below 25). Professionals in the field of mental retardation have included the criterion of adaptive behavior in the definition of mental retardation because an IQ score alone does not reveal the particular living, working, or leisure skills possessed by an individual. There is much behavioral variability among different individuals who have similar IQ scores, due to such factors as individual learning histories and different environmental opportunities. In fact, the behavioral variability exhibited by retarded persons of similar IQ scores, and the effect of the environment on this variability, has caused some professionals to argue that mental retardation is best conceptualized as a *role* played by a person rather than simply a syndrome of symptoms or characteristics.[7] Specifically, mildly retarded persons are often not considered to be mentally retarded in all of the environments in which they function. For example, a mildly retarded youngster might attend special education classes but upon graduation, he or she might obtain competitive employment and, in the vocational role, no longer bear the label of mental retardation. The extent to which mentally retarded persons continue to be identified as mentally retarded during the time that they are elderly is a matter for empirical investigation. It may be that the differences between older mentally retarded persons and older persons in general are not as large as when both groups were younger. The social roles played by elderly persons are less competitive and less exacting than those played by adults prior to old age. Thus, retarded persons—especially those with mild retardation—might function more similarly to normal persons during this period in life, especially if they have not been socialized too strongly to the "retarded" role.

Another important component of the definition of mental retardation is age of onset. As noted above, the AAMD definition uses the words "manifested during the developmental period" to refer to the period from birth through 18 years. The purpose of this definitional component is to differentiate between childhood and adult onset of cognitive and adaptive behavior impairments. Thus, although some elderly persons who have mental status problems and who have problems carrying out activities of daily living might behave in a fashion similar to some mentally retarded persons, the criterion of age of onset is critical in distinguishing between the two population groups.

Using the AAMD definition, approximately 3% of the population is classified as mentally retarded. The vast majority (over 95%) of retarded persons live in noninstitutional settings and attend school or hold jobs. Over 90% are classified in the mild and moderate range. For most, the etiology of their retardation is unknown.

Size of the Elderly Mentally Retarded Population

How many elderly mentally retarded persons are there in the United States? Although no direct epidemiological study of this population has been conducted, it is possible to make estimates based on available data and projections. According to *The Chartbook on Aging in America* prepared for the 1981 White House Conference on Aging, in 1980 11.2% of the United States population was over the age of 65 and another 9.6% was between the ages of 55 and 64.[8] Together, these two categories included 46 million persons. Applying estimates of the prevalence of mental retardation to these data, it becomes possible to estimate the number of mentally retarded elderly in 1980. Using the AAMD's estimate of 3% of the population, there are approximately 1,380,000 mentally retarded persons over the age of 55 in the United States. However, some authors have asserted that mentally retarded persons have a shorter lifespan than nonretarded persons, and therefore they argue that the use of the 3% prevalence estimate is inaccurate. O'Connor, Justice, & Warren[9] estimated that the mentally retarded constitute only 2.4% of the elderly population due to early deaths. Using this prevalence estimate, there were approximately 1,104,000 mentally retarded persons over the age of 55 in the United States in 1980. Thus, it is likely that the mentally retarded elderly range in number from roughly 1 million one hundred thousand to close to 1 million four hundred thousand.

Using these estimates, it is clear that the subgroup of elderly mentally retarded persons is large, and is likely to be growing in size in the future because the absolute number of elderly persons is increasing as the population in general increases, and because the life span of mentally retarded persons in particular is increasing because of improvements in medical care received by them. Seen from another perspective, the size of the general population which is *affected* by mental retardation among persons over the age of 55—either directly or as the aging parents, siblings, or other relatives of older retarded persons—is very large, at least several million persons.

Although little has been written about the service needs of elderly mentally retarded persons or their families, it is probable that a large proportion will at some time need services from social workers. Roles filled by social workers include arranging for guardianship and protective services, counseling relatives of elderly mentally retarded clients and the elderly mentally retarded clients themselves, coordinating services, advocating for increased access to services, etc. Thus, the elderly mentally retarded and their families can be seen as a recently identified subgroup requiring and receiving social work intervention.

THE ELDERLY MENTALLY RETARDED: A PROFILE

Residential Status

Information about the residential status of elderly mentally retarded persons is somewhat limited. Most mentally retarded persons live in the community, either with relatives, friends, or alone. No more than 5% of the general mentally retarded population has ever been institutionalized. Today, because of deinstitutionalization, the percentage is considerably smaller. The literature does not indicate whether the proportion of mentally retarded who are elderly and who reside in institutions is higher or lower than 5%. The increased need of this subgroup for long-term residential services, as compared with younger mentally retarded clients, would suggest the possibility of a higher rate of institutional living among the aged retarded, although the percentage might also be affected by the higher death rate of severely and profoundly retarded persons who constitute the majority of the institutionalized mentally retarded population. Hill, Lakin, Sigford, Hauber, and Bruininks[10] surveyed community residences and institutions serving mentally retarded persons in 1977 and 1978 and reported that the percentage of clients over age 51 was somewhat greater in institutions than in community residences (14% vs. 11%, respectively). However, no information about the much larger group of elderly mentally retarded persons who live independently or with relatives in the community is available from this study. Neuman[11] reported that approximately one-third of the residents of Letchworth Village (an institution in New York State) were over age 55, a much higher percentage than that reported by Hill et al.

It is possible that over time, access to community residential placements for older mentally retarded persons has increased. A study conducted in the early 1970's[12] reported that approximately 7% of the residents of community residences in operation at that time were over the age of 51. A comparison of this finding with the Hill et al. data reported above suggests that the proportion of elderly mentally retarded clients in community residences may be increasing over time. This client group also tends to move less rapidly than younger mentally retarded adults from community residences to more independent living arrangements, and thus may occupy a larger and larger proportion of the beds in community residences as time passes.

Several other studies provide interesting data about the types of community residences in which elderly mentally retarded persons are placed. Seltzer, Seltzer, and Sherwood[13] compared deinstitutionalized retarded adults aged 54 and below with those aged 55 and above, and reported significant differences in the living arrangements of these two groups. Whereas 18% of the younger group lived in their own apartments, not a single one of the older group did so. In contrast, 68% of the older group lived in foster homes, as compared with only 15% of the younger group. Bruininks and his colleagues[14] also reported a higher percentage of older mentally retarded persons living in foster homes as compared with group homes.

In the placement of mentally retarded persons in residential settings, it is possible that different age groups prefer different living arrangements. Sweeney and Wilson reported that 18 of 23 institutionalized elderly mentally retarded persons whom they interviewed "emphatically" wished to stay in the institution. The average length of institutionalization of this group was 38 years. The authors conclude by recommending:

> We have the responsibility to ensure a safe, secure, dignified living for the well aged. This must be provided taking into consideration their long life history. If this happens to be in an institution, we must not feel guilty. We cannot be held accountable for what was done 40 years ago—we must not become guilty by taking them out now if this is the best place. . .[15]

As will be discussed in greater detail later in this chapter, central issues concerning the residential status of elderly mentally retarded persons are stability and permanence. In order to maximize these ends, social workers can assist families in the development of guardianship plans for the aging mentally retarded individual. Additionally, social workers may be very valuable to families in helping them to accept the reality that a secure, permanent residential placement may be impossible to insure absolutely, and instead to motivate family members to remain involved with their elderly mentally retarded relative on an ongoing basis to monitor the quality and appropriateness of the residential placement.

Health Status

Only a few systematic investigations have been conducted about the health status of the population of elderly mentally retarded persons. Callison et al.[16] conducted an interesting study which compared elderly mentally retarded, elderly schizophrenic, and elderly normal persons with respect to changes in their visual ability, hearing, and grip strength. All groups were found to deteriorate over time in these three areas. However, among the three groups, the mentally retarded elderly deteriorated most in vision and hearing. Thus, with respect to sensory activities, it may be that the combination of advanced age and mental retardation poses special problems.

In several other studies, direct or indirect comparisons were made between elderly mentally retarded persons and nonretarded elderly persons, or between younger and older retarded adults. Anglin[17] reported the findings of a survey of 28 mentally retarded adults over the age of 50. A family practice physician was asked to evaluate the health status of these clients and compare them with the general nonretarded elderly population. The physician concluded that while the health problems of older mentally retarded persons were typical of the elderly population in general, the elderly mentally retarded were more likely to have seizure disorders and hearing problems and less likely to have heart problems and high blood pressure. Seltzer, Sherwood, and Sherwood[18] reported on the health status of a group of mentally retarded persons averaging 53 years of age. Seizure disorders, Parkinson's, multiple sclerosis, and lung diseases were noted as special health problems.

In another study, Seltzer et al.[19] examined the characteristics of older and younger deinstitutionalized mentally retarded adults and found that the two groups were comparable in the number of health problems that had been recorded in the institution's records prior to the client's deinstitutionalization. However, comparability in *number* of health problems does not necessarily imply comparability in *severity* of health problems, and thus it is possible that the older group was in fact more debilitated than the younger group. It is also possible that the effects of long years of institutionalization on the health of these clients masked differences between the two groups which otherwise might have been evident.

Neuman[20] reported that as many as 27% of the residents of Letchworth Village who were over age 55 required skilled nursing care. At first glance this appears to be a strikingly high rate, in view of the fact that only approximately 5% of the nonretarded elderly population receives nursing home care. However, Neuman's clients may not be at all typical of the older mentally retarded population. Since the sample was still institutionalized in an era when the pressure to deinstitutionalize was great, it is possible that this residual group had an unusually high rate of health problems.

Together, these studies offer only a very limited knowledge base about the health status of older mentally retarded adults. However, several general guidelines are suggested that may be useful in social work practice with this client population. First, more frequent health screening and more vigilant medical monitoring might be advisable for this group than for the general elderly population, due to the possibility of a more rapid deterioration in their sensory abilities and neurological and neuromuscular disorders. Second, extra medical care might be necessary for elderly mentally retarded clients who have had long years of institutionalization.

While older mentally retarded persons may have more or less severe mental health problems than the elderly in general, the majority were not found to pose unusual or special medical management challenges. Although the more severe the retardation the more likely that an individual has a physiological reason for retardation, a relatively small proportion of mentally retarded persons are severely and profoundly retarded. Even among Down's Syndrome adults, who are believed to have a higher than normal incidence of Alzheimer's disease, the way that this disease is manifested does not appear to be atypical. Thus, with the exception of some severely and profoundly retarded clients who have special syndromes, generic health services are advisable for most elderly mentally retarded clients. One challenge facing social workers is obtaining access to generic health services for this underserved population.

Functional Status

Gerontologists agree that a key difference between elderly and younger adults in the general population is that the elderly function at a lower level with respect to many activities of daily living. Seltzer et al.[21] reported that the older group in their sample were found to function at a significantly lower level of independence than the younger group of retarded adults in the sample even though the two groups were comparable in intellectual level (IQ scores). Although there is generally a positive correlation between functional abilities and IQ scores, it is possible that as retarded persons age, other factors such as health status and availability of services may have a negative impact on their functional abilities.

A related issue pertains to the decline in intellectual capacity with age. Very little is known about this issue with respect to the mentally retarded population; however, two studies which attempted to trace changes in intellectual capacity over time failed to find decreases in IQ scores among older mentally retarded sample members.[22]

The intellectual and functional domains are related to one another in a complex manner. However, practitioners should give primary attention to the functional domain. The quality of life of clients will be negatively affected to a much greater degree by diminishing functional abilities than by diminishing intellectual abilities. Similarly, family members of elderly mentally retarded persons—who have had many years to adjust to the impaired intellectual abilities of the retarded person—may justifiably become alarmed if their retarded relatives begin to fail to perform skills that they had previously mastered. Along with changes in health status, declining functioning abilities may be a prime antecedent to the placement of elderly mentally retarded persons in long-term care settings. Thus, an important role for social workers who have older mentally retarded clients is to help arrange for the provision of services and the structuring of environments that will maximize the maintenance of functional skills.

In sum, more research on elderly mentally retarded persons is sorely needed. Very few practice articles about this group have been published, perhaps reflecting the current lack of services provided to them. It is difficult to confidently generalize practice principles from the limited amount of work that is available because the study samples are often atypical and few attempts to replicate the findings have been made.

However, in the section that follows, an attempt will be made to identify key problems affecting this group. Some of these problems are unique to the elderly retarded and others are shared with elderly persons in general. All of these problems may require the intervention of a social worker.

SPECIAL PROBLEMS
OF THE ELDERLY MENTALLY RETARDED

Parental Aging and Death

Primary among the problems faced by the elderly mentally retarded is the aging and death of their parents. As discussed earlier in this chapter, the family is often a retarded person's best resource, providing advocacy, training, and support. However, elderly retarded persons generally do not have as many family resources upon which to draw as do younger retarded persons. As parents age, their capacity to act on the behalf of their adult-aged or elderly retarded child diminishes considerably. This is especially true for families who may have placed their retarded child in an institution, as ties are generally weakened as a result of institutionalization.

Parental aging may precipitate a crisis for the retarded son or daughter. Who will replace the parents as natural allies and advocates? It is rare for elderly retarded persons to have had children who can assume responsibility for them in later life. The retarded person's siblings may be called upon to fill this role. However, siblings and other relatives are often ambivalent about their assuming this responsibility. They are aging also, have their own families and needs, and may have many conflicting emotions about their retarded relative including anger and guilt as well as love. They may also fear that the retarded person might become a financial burden for the relative. For all of these reasons the relatives may need help in coping. As Adams[23] pointed out, the objective of the casework relationship with families of retarded persons is "bolstering them up as they mobilize their resources for the long emotional and practical siege that is involved in caring for a retarded. . . relative" (p. 158).

Another problem provoked by parental aging and death is the adjustment of the older mentally retarded person to the death of a parent. This is especially problematic when the retarded person has lived at home throughout his or her life. Often there is a very strong interdependence between parent and adult-aged child, and at times, there is an overdependence on both of their parts. The retarded person may be infantalized by the parent, and thus may have more limited skills and maturity than he or she might otherwise have developed. The adult retarded son or daughter may demand a degree of physical and psychological involvement from the parent not at all commensurate with actual need. When the parent dies, this relationship is abruptly severed. Although parental death often provokes adjustment reactions in "normal" adult-aged children, when the son or daughter is mentally retarded, the special nature and intensity of the parent-child relationship may make the adjustment even more difficult. In addition, cognitive limitations and emotional immaturity may further complicate an already difficult situation.

The following case illustrates many of the problems faced by an older retarded person whose parent is aging.

Frank, age 63, is a mentally retarded man who lives with his mother and his brother, George. Neither brother has ever left home. George is paraplegic, unemployed, and often depressed. Their mother, Mrs. B is in her 80's, and has recently deteriorated cognitively and physically. She attends a daycare program for the elderly, but her increasing senility may limit how much longer she can remain in this program.

The social worker is currently working with Frank around the issue of placing his mother in a nursing home. Frank is extremely upset about this prospect, since taking care of his mother has become such a strong part of his identity.

What will happen to Frank when Mrs. B is placed in the nursing home? There is no extended family. Frank's brother George cannot provide financial or emotional support. How Frank will adjust to the loss of his mother is unclear. Her absence could precipitate a major emotional crisis for Frank.

In sum, then, special problems are posed by the aging and death of parents of older mentally retarded adults. First, it is often the case that the separation that usually occurs between adults and their parents has failed to be effected when the son or daughter is mentally retarded. In such cases, the retarded person's emotional adjustment following the death of a parent might be very difficult. In addition, when the parent dies, the retarded adult loses a natural advocate at a time when the need for advocacy may be increasing. Relatives, who may be called upon to assume responsibility, may have ambivalent feelings about this role or may be unable to do so. The social worker can provide support critical to the well-being of all involved during this difficult time.

Social Isolation

A related problem is social isolation. Older mentally retarded persons often have diminished informal support systems, as friends and family members age. Similarly, the formal support system provides considerably fewer social opportunities to elderly retarded persons than to younger retarded adults. Access to sheltered workshops, special social groups, community residences and other services often becomes more difficult as a retarded person ages.

Another problem is that existing friendship groups may be broken up. It is relatively uncommon for a group of retarded persons who were friends in the institution to be placed in the same geographic area in the community following deinstitutionalization. This problem often is exacerbated when older retarded persons are forced to move from one community to another in order to live with or be near to a member of the family. Friends are left behind, and it may become increasingly difficult with age to make new friends. The social isolation that is characteristic of many nonretarded elderly persons is thus even more likely to occur among the retarded elderly.

One strategy to combat social isolation among the elderly retarded is the formation of special social groups and programs for them. These programs differ from programs for younger retarded adults in that they tend to place a lower priority on achievement and the mastery of new skills than on leisure time activities and the maintenance of functional abilities. Although there are many advantages to special programs for the elderly mentally retarded, such as increased access and more specialized activities, there are also disadvantages. Some professionals have argued that the segregation of retarded persons in special programs may have unintended negative consequences. As Mahoney[24] has cautioned:

> It becomes all too easy. . . to isolate deviants and to ease them into compartmentalized activities in the name of providing special programs to meet their needs. Because it is easier,

however, because it is more comfortable, because it is more administratively efficient, does not mean it is better. . . .

An alternative to special programs is the integration of elderly retarded persons into programs for elderly persons in general. This is the implementation of the normalization principle, which encourages:

> making available to the mentally retarded patterns and conditions of everyday life which are as close as possible to norms and patterns of the mainstream of society.[25]

An example of such integration is the placement of an elderly retarded woman with a group of cognitively impaired nonretarded elderly in a day care center. Another example of the use of generic services is two elderly retarded men in an apartment unit in a federally subsidized apartment building for the elderly. Integration of elderly retarded persons into generic programs typically requires a considerable amount of prior advocacy on the part of the social worker and vigilant monitoring on an ongoing basis once the placement is made. Not only must the social worker focus on problems of initial access, it is also necessary to work with the program staff in order to educate them about the needs of the client and the most appropriate methods of interacting with and involving him or her in the group. In addition, the elderly mentally retarded client often needs support in rising to the challenge of and adapting to an integrated experience. Since it is possible to feel isolated even in an integrated situation, it may be preferable for several elderly mentally retarded persons to be involved in a program simultaneously rather than including only one such person. Perhaps most difficult, the social worker might need to meet with the nonretarded elderly persons who participate in the program if they have negative feelings about the integration of retarded persons into their group. The stigma of mental retardation can be particularly threatening to persons who are anxious about their own cognitive capacities and ability to function competently.

To sum up, social isolation is a problem of particular importance to retarded persons during their old age. In general, elderly mentally retarded persons are not seen as highly desirable clients either by gerontology programs, which generally serve the "normal" elderly, or by mental retardation programs, which generally serve younger retarded persons. Sometimes integrating the elderly mentally retarded in with one of these two general groups is preferable, while at other times the elderly retarded person benefits more from placement into a special social group. The preferences of the retarded person, the existence of resources, and the availability of the natural support system of the retarded person all have an influence on the extent to which social isolation is a problem in an individual case. Supportive social work interventions including advocacy by the social worker are often critical in helping the elderly mentally retarded person to cope with this problem.

Need for Permanency Planning

The vulnerability of elderly mentally retarded persons—physically, socially, cognitively—and the increasingly limited resources available to them may precipitate crises of care and adjustment. The effects of such crises may be minimized if families do careful advance planning.

Permanency planning is often used in foster care services to children. It involves the development of a plan which has as its goal the placement of a foster child into a permanent home—a home in which the child can live until he or she reaches adulthood. By extension, permanency planning can offer a useful perspective on social work practice with elderly mentally retarded persons. Plans can be developed which have as their goal insuring as secure a lifestyle as possible for the elderly retarded person until he or she dies. As Begab and Goldberg[26] explain:

> Parents of normal children generally can look forward to the time when their children will achieve some measure of financial security and social prestige. For many of the retarded, however, . . . these are unattainable goals. For those among the retarded who are chronically dependent or semi-dependent persons, a lifetime plan of guidance, care, and supervision is needed.

Permanency planning does not result in an unchangeable plan, but rather a plan that will be in force until it is amended. Such plans for mentally retarded individuals often include three components: resi-

dential security, legal protection, and financial security. Each will
be briefly discussed below.

Some families are eager to make plans which insure that the aging
mentally retarded person will have a secure place to live until he or
she dies, but do not know how to go about creating such a plan. In
contrast, other families are reluctant to discuss the possibility that a
time will come when the parents are no longer able to care for their
adult-aged retarded child. Social workers can make an important
contribution to both of these types of family through casework intervention by helping them to acknowledge this difficult problem
and to begin to make appropriate plans. Still other types of families
have distanced themselves from their retarded family member,
often following institutionalization. Years later and often with great
ambivalence, many families have attempted to reconnect with their
adult-aged retarded children who have since been placed in the community. Casework around the issue of the future residential security
of the retarded adult is perhaps the most challenging with these
families because once before—usually upon the advice of professionals—they had attempted to arrange a secure residential placement for their retarded child in the institution, and have since been
told—again by professionals—that the arrangement they chose is
neither appropriate nor will it provide a lifelong home.

Although private residential facilities are often prohibitively expensive and generally do not insure permanence beyond the time
that funding for the resident is available, families who do have sufficient funds can consider this option. One type of private residential
facility is the sheltered village, which provides a self-contained separate community for retarded persons. As Baker, Seltzer, and
Seltzer[27] described:

> Common to all sheltered villages is the segregation of the
> retarded person . . . from the outside community, and the im-
> plicit view that the retarded adult is better off living in an envi-
> ronment that shelters him or her from many of the potential
> failures and frustrations of life in the outside community. . .

The trade-off made when a family places an adult son or daughter in
a sheltered village is limited opportunities to encounter new experiences and to take risks in return for insuring security and a sense of
community. The social worker can help the family to consider the

appropriateness of this decision and to help them select the option that seems to be in the retarded person's best interest.

A second component of permanency planning for elderly retarded persons is legal protection. Boggs[28] pointed out that social service agencies have traditionally provided protective services to children. Protective services, which she defines as "social services directed toward the welfare of individuals who are not fully able to act for themselves" (p. 593), are only minimally provided by agencies to adults even though some disabled adults and elderly persons may be as vulnerable as minors. Some mentally retarded persons, especially elderly mentally retarded persons, need assistance in money management and making important decisions. In such cases, guardians may be appointed by the courts. The guardian can serve as the retarded person's advocate and can attempt to protect him or her from exploitation. Parents normally fill this role, but, as was pointed out above, as parents age their capacity to function in this role generally diminishes. In preparation for such a time, some parents appoint a testamentary guardian for their retarded son or daughter. This is a person who will assume responsibility for the retarded person when the parents die.

Many persons may be involved in the decision to establish guardianship: the judge, the lawyer, the guardian, the social worker, the family, and the retarded person. The social worker can provide support to the retarded person and the family as the plans for another person to take over the affairs of the retarded son or daughter are evaluated. There are some instances in which the family perceives that the retarded older person is in need of a guardian, but professional opinion may believe that he or she could successfully manage independently. In such cases, the social worker can help the family recognize that their mentally retarded relative is competent in spite of his or her age and mental retardation.

The third component of a permanent plan for an older retarded person involves financial security. There are many obvious reasons why arranging for as much security as possible in this area is very important. First and foremost, there is the welfare of the retarded person. In addition, the relatives and/or guardian may not be in a position to assume all of the financial burden of the retarded person. While a few families will be able to leave an estate sufficiently large to cover all or most of the costs incurred by or on behalf of their retarded son or daughter, most will not be in this position. An alternative source of financial security is Supplemental Security Income (SSI) for which most mentally retarded persons are eligible. SSI, which is accompanied by Medicaid benefits, provides a modest but regular income that can constitute or form a component of a permanent financial plan for the elderly retarded person.

In sum, there are three key components of permanency planning for elderly mentally retarded persons: residential security, legal protection, and financial security. The extent to which any family and/or retarded person needs the support and expertise of a social worker in arranging for each of these components varies from case to case, depending upon the capacities and resources of the retarded person and the family. Often, however, some professional intervention is desirable in order to minimize anxiety about the future and to maximize the extent to which the family can provide support in as reliable a fashion as possible, so that the retarded person can face a secure old age. The following case illustrates these points.

Mrs. H., a widow in her 70's, has two sons in their 50's. Jerry, who is mentally retarded, was adopted at the age of nine. When he was adopted, he had severe behavior problems and very limited language and self-care skills. Sam is two years younger than Jerry.

Today, Jerry functions in the mildly retarded range. He can read and write, holds a volunteer job, shops, runs errands, and can do minor household repairs. However, he is quite dependent upon his mother for supervision and guidance in all of these activities.

Mrs. H. is well-off financially. Jerry has never held a paying job, primarily because of his secure financial status. In her will, Mrs. H. stipulated that her son Sam, who lives in another city, will inherit her house and that Jerry will continue to live there indefinitely. Jerry will inherit his mother's money. With the support of the family's social worker, Sam has agreed to become Jerry's guardian. Since Sam and Jerry have a good relationship, the expectation is that these arrangements will work out.

Will Jerry be able to live independently after Mrs. H. dies? He would need to learn to perform independently many community survival skills. With training, he probably could improve his functional abilities. Mrs. H. is reluctant to allow him to receive such training. Loneliness might also be a problem.

Although he has friends, he rarely brings them home because Mrs. H. disapproves of many of them. The family's social worker is currently working with Mrs. H. to encourage her to allow Jerry to receive training in the area of independent performance of functional skills before she dies and to allow him to bring his friends home more freely at the present time.

Social work intervention in this case is intended to create a more secure plan for Jerry's future once his mother dies. The social worker first mobilized the brother to become Jerry's guardian and is currently working with the mother to permit Jerry to become more independent socially and functionally. Successful resolution of this issue will maximize the extent to which Jerry's future is secure.

SUMMARY AND CONCLUSIONS

In conclusion, a number of social work practice issues have been identified that pertain to the population of elderly mentally retarded persons. First, in the residential domain, there is a need for social workers to mobilize family members to help them make or reaffirm a long-term commitment to monitoring the quality and appropriateness of the living arrangement of their elderly mentally retarded relative. The field of mental retardation has long been characterized by successful advocacy by family members in securing and monitoring services. However, it is generally young adult or middle-aged parents who advocate for the needs of their younger retarded children. The challenge of mobilizing very elderly parents, siblings, or more distant relatives such as nephews/nieces to become involved in the coordination of services for an elderly retarded relative is a much more difficult task.

Second, it appears that the elderly mentally retarded generally do not have highly specialized health care needs. Thus, the challenge facing social workers is to advocate for increased access for older mentally retarded persons to generic health services. Given the negative attitudes held by society in general toward both the mentally retarded and the elderly, easy access to these and other services cannot be assumed. Family members and the older mentally retarded clients themselves will need support and strategic assistance in their attempts to arrange for high quality services.

Third, in the functional domain, there is a need for social workers to advocate for the provision of a service package which maximizes the probability that elderly mentally retarded clients will maintain their functional abilities to the greatest extent possible. This includes obtaining prosthetic devices, adapting the home environment, and arranging for sensory stimulation as needed in order to enable the older mentally retarded person to retain as independent a lifestyle as possible.

Fourth, families often need help in making future plans for the older retarded person in order to maximize his or her financial, legal, and residential security. Social workers have substantive expertise in permanency planning that can be applied to this client population. Furthermore, they can help the family to address issues that otherwise might not be discussed directly because they raise complex emotions among those involved. Thus, permanency planning involves both arranging for concrete services and supportive interventions.

The provision of support to families and to elderly mentally retarded persons is an important role for social workers with respect to all of the issues discussed in this chapter. Each issue poses challenges that may provoke family or individual crises or otherwise prompt the need for intervention. Adjustments to shifting family responsibilities, declining health, and diminished functional abilities not only require instrumental responses on the part of those involved but also reaching a new emotional equilibrium. In dealing with this clinical challenge, social work intervention can often be critical to the successful resolution of problems.

In sum, the activities which need to be performed by social workers in providing services to the elderly mentally retarded and their families are diverse, ranging from clinical intervention to advocacy to case management and coordination. Although some unique information about mental retardation is needed, social workers can draw on their existing framework of knowledge, values, and skills in providing services to this group of clients. This is especially true with respect to the mildly retarded who constitute the vast majority of the mentally retarded group. As Dickerson[29] pointed out:

> The role and responsibilities of a caseworker with a mentally retarded client are unique only because of the retardation. The social worker must perceive his role in relation to such a client just as he would in any other client relationship: he has the responsiblity to understand retardation, even as a worker in

another setting would need to understand gerontology or alcoholism.

REFERENCES

1. Lowy, L. *Social Policies and programs on aging*. Lexington: Lexington Books, 1980.
    Monk, A. Social Work with the aged: Principles of Practice. *Social Work*, 1981, 26, 61-68.
    2. Baker, B.L., Seltzer, B.G., & Seltzer, M.M. *As close as possible: Community residences for retarded adults*. Boston: Little, Brown, 1977.
    Talkington, L.W. & Chiovaro, S.J. An approach to programming for aged MR. *Mental Retardation*, 1969, 7, 29-30.
    3. Neuman, F. Ready, set go—The institutionalized aging and aged developmentally disabled client: A new look at an old topic. Paper presented at the Annual Conference of the American Association on Mental Deficiency, June, 1981.
    Seltzer, M.M., Seltzer, G.B., & Sherwood, C.C. Comparison of Community Adjustment of older vs. younger mentally retarded adults. *American Journal of Mental Deficiency*, 1982, 87, 9-13.
    4. O'Connor, G., Justice, R.S., & Warren, N. The aged mentally retarded: Institution or community care? *American Journal of Mental Deficiency*, 1970, 75, 354-360.
    Sherwood, S. & Gruenberg, L. *A descriptive study of functionally eligible applicants to the Domiciliary Care Program*. Boston: Hebrew Rehabilitation Center for Aged, unpublished manuscript, 1979.
    5. Tymchuk, A.J. The mentally retarded in later life. *In* Kaplan, O.J. (ed.), *Psychopathology of Aging*. N.Y.: Academic Press, 1979.
    6. Grossman, H. *Manual on Terminology and Classification*. Washington, D.C.: American Association on Mental Deficiency, 1977, p.11.
    7. Mercer, J. *Labelling the Mentally Retarded: Clinical and social system perspectives on mental retardation*. Berkeley: University of California Press, 1973.
    8. Allan, C. & Brotman, H. *Chartbook on aging in America*. White House Conference on Aging, 1981.
    9. O'Connor, Justice & Warren, op. cit.
    10. Hill, B.K., Lakin, K.C., Sigford, B.B., Hauber, F.A., & Bruininks, R.H. *Programs and services for mentally retarded people in residential facilities*. Minneapolis: University of Minnesota, 1982.
    11. Neuman, F., op. cit.
    12. O'Connor, G. *Home is a good place: a national perspective of community residential facilities for developmentally disabled persons*. Washington, D.C: American Association on Mental Deficiency, 1976.
    13. Seltzer, Seltzer & Sherwood, op. cit.
    14. Bruininks, R.H., Hauber, F.A. & Kudla, M.J. *National Survey of community residential facilities: A profile of facilities and residents in 1977*. (Project report No. 5) Minneapolis: University of Minnesota, 1979.
    Bruininks, R.H., Hill, B. & Thorsheim, M.J. *A profile of specially licensed foster homes for mentally retarded people in 1977*. (Project report No. 6) Minneapolis: University of Minnesota, 1980.
    15. Sweeney, D.P., Wilson, T.Y. (eds.) *Double Jeopardy: The plight of aging and aged developmentally disabled persons in Mid-America*. Ann Arbor: University of Michigan, 1979, p.22.
    16. Callison, D.A., Armstron, H.F., Elam, L., Cannon, R.L., Paisley, C.M. & Himwich, H. The effects of aging on schizophrenic and mentally defective patients: Visual, auditory and grip strength measurements. *Journal of Gerontology*, 1971, 26, 137-145.

17. Anglin, B. *They never asked for help: A study of the needs of elderly retarded people in Metro Toronto.* Maple, Ontario: Belsten Publishing Co., 1981.
18. Seltzer, M.M., Sherwood, C.C., & Sherwood, S. *A study of the adjustive behavior of placed domiciliary care residents.* Boston: Hebrew Rehabilitation Center for Aged, unpublished manuscript, 1981.
19. Seltzer, Seltzer & Sherwood, op. cit.
20. Neuman, op. cit.
21. Seltzer, Seltzer & Sherwood, op. cit.
22. Bell, A. & Zubek, J.P. The effect of age in the intellectual performance of mental defectives. *Journal of Gerontology*, 1960, 15, 285-295.
Jarvik, L.F. & Falek, A. Intellectual stability and survival in the aged. *Journal of Gerontology*, 1963, 18, 173-176.
23. Adams, M. *Mental retardation and its social dimensions.* N.Y.: Columbia University Press, 1971.
24. Mahoney, S.C. Special community programs for the mildly retarded: Acceptance or rejection? In Schreiber, M. (ed.) *Social Work and Mental Retardation.* N.Y.: John Day, 1970, p.264.
25. Nirje, B. The normalizaton principle and its human management implications, In Kugel, R.B. & Wolfensberger, W. (eds.) *Changing patterns in residential services for the mentally retarded.* Washington, D.C.: President's Committee on Mental Retardation, 1969, p.181.
26. Begab, M.J. & Goldberg, H.L. Guardianship for the mentally retarded, In Schreiber, M. (ed.) *Social Work and Mental Retardation.* N.Y.: John Day, 1970, p.586.
27. Baker, Seltzer & Seltzer, op. cit., p.109.
28. Boggs, E.M. The need for protective services for the mentally retarded and others with serious long-term disabilities. In Schreiber, M. (ed.) *Social Work and Mental Retardation.* N.Y.: John Day, 1970.
29. Dickerson, M.U. *Social Work Practice with the mentally retarded.* New York: The Free Press, 1981, p.146.

Chapter VIII

Permanent Patients:
On Working With
the Chronic Mentally Frail
in the Community

David Feldstein

Shambly man.
Tousled, troubled, old man
What are you about?

Strollers, a wide berth give
Denying by stare, your birth.
Asking themselves
"Why are you here? Why are you?"
Answering
"Promenade elsewhere, taking your life with you."

"Do not remind us,
    What we may yet be."

INTRODUCTION

Many elderly persons have become permanent patients. One group, to whom a large body of literature and study is devoted, are in nursing homes or other protected settings.[1] Generally they comprise between 5 and 10% of the population over 65.[2] A walk in any urban, and many suburban communities reveals a highly visible population of troubled (and to some observers, troublesome) persons,[3] confirming the view that many in need of mental health services are not in institutions.[4] This chapter describes some of the conditions which have helped create this new underclass, its parameters, and its constituents. Strategies of service for a selected group, the mentally frail and ill elderly, will be examined.

Social Etiology

Of the many ongoing changes in our society, three in particular have come together to impact on the elderly over the last decade or so. First, is the changing perception and use of the psychiatric hospital; second the increase in life expectancy; and, third, the mobility of younger generations combined with dramatic changes in the urban housing stock.*

Views of the psychiatric hospital started to change after 1950 with the introduction of phenothiazines. In following years, a virtual armamentarium of psychoactive pharmaceuticals have been introduced.[5] The interior of the hospital became a subject of study,[6] as did the impact of institutionalization as a socializing force.[7] It became clear that institutions were neither necessarily ennobling nor humane, nor even benign.[8] "Warehouse" rather than hospital became a definiens. Particularly after 1963 with the passage of the Community Mental Health Centers Act,[9] questioning of the value of prolonged hospitalization emerged. We then started to release, or to some, "remove," persons no longer in need of ongoing care. The deinstitutionalization movement, once underway, has resulted in a most dramatic decline in long term psychiatric hospitalization.[10] This took place at about the same time that the large increase in nursing homes started under the impetus of the Medicare/Medicaid provisions of the Social Security Act.[11] For many, deinstitutionalization meant reinstitutionalization.[12] Funding shifted to largely federal sources. The economic rationale** on a State level underpinned a civil rights and humanitarian strategy.*** The growth of the population of those over 65 with no corresponding growth in hospital beds also served to constrict admissions.[13]

Concurrently, psychiatric hospitals have moved to admit only the acutely ill. In some instances, this has just meant the homicidal or suicidal.[14] The hospital is no longer a place of refuge. Population

---

*This list is hardly exhaustive. The three to which attention are primarily paid provide a context. A fourth factor is also noted in passing, viz., negative attitudes towards and stereotypes of, the elderly. In addition, many events also impinge upon the mental health of the elderly. Financial fears, acts of discrimination, physical disability, the death of a spouse or a child, and a cut back in entitlements, are only suggestive of the range.

**I.e., Medicare and Medicaid, exclusive or largely Federal programs, do not pay for prolonged psychiatric hospitalization, but Medicaid will support life-long care in a nursing home.

***The failure of States and localities to provide planned community services is only noted in passing.

(i.e., possible patients) was thus lost by both admission and discharge policies.

It is in vogue to apply much of the same language of frustration to the nursing home.[15] We see this most clearly in the expression, "alternatives to institutionalization." The deinstitutionalization movement has simultaneously occurred in State Schools. The same forces affect this population also. A growing group of the elderly mentally retarded are in need of services though they are not the primary focus of this paper.

People are also living longer. Life expectancy is now 68.7 for men and 76.5 for women. (Men who reach 65 can expect to live 13 more years, women 18.) Indeed, in the last several years we have begun to see references to the young-old and the old-old.[16] The latter being the most rapidly growing segment of our population.[17]

Finally, the suburbs and the cities are in flux. The former are older and often need rebuilding, capital infusion, amenities, and social services. Their aging is strongly reflected by increasing numbers of empty classrooms. Earlier on, the flight to the suburbs left a residual, aging population in the cities. They are still there. However, there has seemingly been an influx of younger persons to the cities. Consequently, an increased pressure on the available housing stock, and a move to upgrade older housing has occurred. Those displaced often are elderly,[18] not viewed as a major target group for neighborhood gentrification.

As always in American history, the society is undergoing change. There is little reason to think that the processes described will, or can be reversed, or even slowed.

Permanent Patients

As a nominative category permanent patients are diverse racially, sexually and ethnically; they cross economic lines; some have families, many are alone or estranged; some may be largely unknown to their neighbors, others call attention to themselves; functional disorders (psychoses) are present; a group are actually or seemingly organically impaired; some are in acute crisis (transient situation disturbances), for others this is a "way of life"; and, some have alcohol or drug problems.[19]

The diversity could be even further extended. However, three characteristics, besides being older, stand out. First, all are mentally disabled, or functioning in some psychological or socially incapacitated way. Next, they are "marginal" in our society. They are not as we wish our own elders to be.[20] Third, they are a stigmatized group, often given the appellation, "crazy." For some, sadly, as in any stigmatized group, the stereotype is adopted as a badge and worn.[21] They blame themselves for things over which they have no control.[22] The devaluation of the old within our society becomes incorporated in their persona.[23]

One significant group are those who have spent some portion of their lives in psychiatric hospitals. "Up until the 1960's in most of the United States, the mental hospital was used as a primary service for old people *whether or not they were mentally ill.*"[24] (emphasis added)

> Miss A. was released from the hospital at age 59 in order to take care of her dying father. She had been a patient for 42 years.

In this example psychiatric hospitalization continued beyond the period of acute need. Miss A. approached old age severely institutionalized. She, like many others, had been released with little preparation for life outside the hospital. Images of the "walking wounded" are often aptly descriptive.[25] No wonder then that they are shunned, becoming objects of public concern and ridicule. They are described as needy as much by their unsightliness as by a humanitarian impulse.[26]

Not every person here dubbed a permanent patient, has a lengthy psychiatric history. A significant number do appear to have had prior contact with psychiatric services on an in or outpatient basis at some time in their lives. Regrettably, good data regarding incidence are not available. Conceptually, this is a loosely defined grouping, almost any psychiatric contact making one fit the definition of "permanent patient."

A critical definiens of the deinstitutionalized and of those who have had prior contact with mental health service of one kind or another is that they were once young mental patients. Now they have become old, and the need for services is reasserted.*

---

*Not every person who has utilized mental health services in younger days is in such need during their older years, of course. That many are, speaks historically as much to the "state of the art" as to the ongoing lack of clarity around "cure," "fully functioning," "remission," etc. The point to be recognized is that "other things being equal" is not truly a phrase of the human condition. There is an element of being "at risk."

Others have lived on the fringes of society a good part of their lives; some have been in good supportive social circumstance. However, some trauma or deteriorative process is evidenced. A "negative disruption" (e.g., eviction, death of a child, institutionalization) occurring without some supportive help could have severe, even tragic, sequelae. This observation highlights the paucity of available, internal resources.

> Mrs. R's "family" were pictures of her deceased husband and son. The former died about ten years earlier; the latter in World War II. She was the last family member alive. Failure to eat regularly added to a presentation of loss and confusion.

And they are generally poor. Surveys note that all the elderly comprise anywhere between one-third and one-fourth of the poor, though they represent only about 11% of the population.[27]

One other common thread is to be noted. They are "survivors."[28] Their ability to survive against the odds already noted, gives credence to the notion that there is a reservoir of strength. This is important diagnostically.

Psychiatry and the Permanent Patient

It seems self-evident that psychiatry would play a large role in the diagnosis and care of these people. Such is not the case, however, though psychiatric nomenclature is widely used. Arnhoff and Kumbar cite the 1970 APA survey noting that 56% of the respondents spent no time with patients over 65 years of age. Of the remainder, 86% spent less than a tenth of their time with elderly patients.[29] Mendenhall's study published in 1978 "indicates that the average psychiatrist spends 5.3% of the total patient care time on patients 65 years of age or older."[30]

Medicare's rather blatant discrimination towards outpatient psychiatry also limits incentive.* Medicaid reimbursement is more liberal, but few psychiatrists are, or necessarily should be, equipped to assist a patient to obtain Medicaid. Psychiatrists who even partially specialize in geriatrics are few. "Geriatric psychiatry is preeminently the field where a multidisciplinary attack is essential in diagnosis, treatment, and placement"[31] notes one observer.[32]

---

*There is a yearly cap of $250 and the psychiatrist is paid at a much lower percentage than other physicians.

The use of psychiatric nosology[33] as a framework speaks strongly to the dominance of medicine, in the diagnosis, if not in the ongoing care of the permanent patient. It also highlights the developed nature of the schema employed, particularly when contrasted with social work formulations.[34] What is here suggested is that psychiatric diagnosis for these patients speaks well to the etiology of the disease processes. It speaks almost as well to the limitations of the patient. However, social work diagnosis, while both less formally structured and developed conceptually, does place a patient in context, highlighting strengths and needs. Thus, for plotting courses of action it is more useful.

Indeed, as Lazarus and Weinberg note in their survey, ". . . the elderly person is usually not referred for psychiatric evaluation until an emergency exists."[35] An optimism has also begun to appear in the psychiatric literature.

> Dramatic improvement of [the patient's] mental state can often be achieved when underlying physical problems are adequately treated, or the patient's milieu is altered so as to receive [as] satisfactory [a] degree of interaction with others as is consistent with the person's life-style.[36]

This even extends to those with organic brain syndromes.[37] Diet, degree of stimulation present or available, and the extent and duration of disruption in a patient's life are all valuable data.

Psychiatry, for all of its development, still wrestles mightily with problems of differential diagnosis. This is nowhere more evident than in work with the elderly.[38] "The risks and discomfort, time and expertise involved, and cost must be weighed against the yield of results that may influence management."[39] The development of the case manager as a viable social work role (and set of tasks) speaks directly to this issue.[40] Equally important to note is that social work is quickly attempting to come to grips with the issues of case management, rather than just noting its problems in passing.

SOCIAL WORK INTERVENTION

The qualifying assumption of the strategies presented is cogently stated by Butler and Lewis, "When in doubt treat and see if improvement occurs."[41] Gurian echoes this. "Active treatment is a most appropriate approach to providing *effective* mental health services for older patients'' [42] (emphasis added).

Three major descriptors of the process—beginnings, stabilization, and linkage—define workers' activities and inform the discussion. The more common term "client" will henceforth be substituted for "patient," to more accurately reflect the social worker as primary to the interventive process.*

Beginnings

This phase of the work may be divided into two separate though often overlapping parts: referral and access. There are few self-referrals. Reaching out to persons with whom potential clients come in contact is more constructive and efficient than trying to locate clients directly. Local merchants, building superintendents, churches and synagogues, the police, landlords, departments of public welfare, social security offices, local organizations and other clients are all useful sources.

Their concern is respected by sharing information about services, quick and courteous response to calls, and, most importantly, a follow up on the intervention. Without violating any confidentiality, one can inform the referrer that engagement has taken place, thank them, and enlist continued help. This enhances an agency's image and furthers its work. The agency must be publicly clear about its responsibility and fealty to the client, as well as its independence and limitations.**

A landlord wanted to refer Mrs. G. who no longer cared for her large and low rental apartment. He was advised that the agency could not support, and might actively fight, eviction. He agreed to introduce the worker to other concerned tenants, who, in turn, helped the worker meet Mrs. G.

This roundabout process prevented any misunderstanding that the social worker was the landlord's worker and helped the agency define an informal support system interested in Mrs. G's welfare.

---

*"Client" is used reluctantly. The connotation of a status differential which adheres to it, makes it less desirable than, e.g., "participant" or "member." These latter terms, unless adjectively modified, impart a stronger sense of mutuality and equality.

**Put another way, the agency's philosophy, policies, and practices must be clearly transmitted to its own staff, as well as to the public.

Referral doesn't always mean ready access. Not all clients want service. Ingenuity and persistence are often needed.

> Mrs. S's family was concerned that she was not eating and becoming a recluse. She wouldn't answer her door. Mr. H., the worker, started leaving cans of a food supplement and soup by her door every other day. He also carried on a monologue about her family's worry and the agency's concern. Several weeks of this activity resulted in the unusual sight of a chair placed outside the door. More weeks passed before they would meet face-to-face.

No attempt, at least initially, to interfere with the psychopathological (paranoid) system at work was made. Effort was directed towards the least threatening engagement. The agency provided a concrete and necessary service (food), which was simultaneously and ultimately nurturing. This is wholly consistent with Goldfarb's dicta about the value and use of dependency.[43] The important thing to be noted is that the work had begun.

> Two referrals of Ms. D. were received within a week. The first was from the police who found her wandering at night; the second from a client who described her as "really crazy." Mrs. T., the worker, made announced visits, but entry was always rebuffed. A fortuitous event intervened, Mrs. T. was in an auto accident and missed five weeks' work. During that time another worker sporadically tried to see Ms. D. The "go-aways" where short and emphatic. Upon returning Mrs. T. again visited the closed door. The response was hostile, but longer. Mrs. T. started to tell Ms. D. when she would be back, but felt dizzy and her voice faltered. Ms. D. said that she hadn't heard what was being said. Mrs. T. apologized saying she felt dizzy. . . the door opened, Ms. D. insisted Mrs. T. come in and sit down, offering her a glass of water.

This poignant example highlights the need for consistency as well as patience. Respect was established by asking if such and such time for the next attempted entry was convenient. Keeping these "appointments" was critical. The growing attachment of Ms. D. to Mrs. T. is seen in the negative reactions to the substitute worker. But, most important, was that Ms. D. wanted and needed contact

and a chance to engage in a reciprocal relationship. The same
dynamic was seen when a chair was placed so Mr. H. could talk
from a more comfortable position. (Mrs. S. had brought her own
chair and sat inside the closed door.) By virtue of expressing a
shared humanity these workers provided the springboard for the
agency to give help.
The above two examples state the difficulty of access with with-
drawn (or withdrawing) clients, but also suggest that it is possible.
Fortunately, such persistence is not always needed, though patience
is.

> Ms. H., who had a spinal condition, took six to eight minutes
> to get to her front door. After the second visit she knew that
> her worker would wait. She no longer had to exhaust herself
> by shouting, asking for patience as she slowly wended her way
> to the door.

> Ms. H., truly a genteel lady, also insisted upon serving tea,
> though this was a painful activity for her. The worker was initially
> uncomfortable with this. However, it became clear that the ritual
> was necessary and supportive of Ms. H.'s social convention; it was
> an intrinsic part of her need to give; and, was indeed part of the pro-
> cess and work.

Stabilization

Conceptually, stabilization is a critical part of the process; discussing it separately is more for intellectual clarity than pragmatic
usage. Three clear, but overlapping purposes are inherent and serve
to guide the work.
Foremost among these, particularly given the frailty, marginality, and often the impaired judgment of these clients, is the need to
prevent further deterioration. As a strategy, then, stabilization is not
to seek immediate improvement, however desirable, but to hinder a
worsening. The case examples already suggest this. With Mrs. S.,
the provision of food was to prevent malnutrition and provide adequate balance in her diet so as to minimize the possibility of her ap-
pearing to have an organic syndrome. The patience and persistence
in her situation as well as with Ms. D. seemed to have worked
against a continuing reclusiveness and paranoid life style.
The second attribute of the stabilization process is that there is a

release of pressure from the client, and often from the agency as well. This is clearly seen with Mrs. G. where the landlord backed off eviction proceedings for several months, giving the agency time to get involved and familiar with her situation. (And, as an aside, with his.) In Mrs. G.'s. situation her "allies" among other tenants also allowed the agency to "cool out" the building. This involved meetings with those who wanted her to remain, as well as with others hostile to her being a neighbor.

The neutralization of conflicting feelings among neighbors is an important stabilizing activity. An agency's conference room can prove to be highly nonthreatening and conducive to problem solving and task sharing.

Ms. D's. friend said, "I'm glad you're here. I'd about run out of patience with her." Her landlord was more explicit, "Good. She's your problem now. I don't know what to do."

The third aspect to be considered is a diagnostic one. As part of the process a working social psychiatric diagnosis is a critical dimension.* Examination of the person and of his environment becomes a part of the stabilization being sought and this examination is not geared toward some set of abstractions, but rather towards a clear and workable understanding. As such this has value with, as well as for, the client.

Intrinsic in a diagnosis[44] is some "looking at" family, friends, and neighbors, or informal support systems. These shall be dealt with in the section on "linkages," *infra*. It is important to note that in the process of discovering "involved others" (truly a diagnostic activity!), they need to be respected, brought into case planning and encouraged to continue, i.e., the agency should not supplant them, but supplement their work and caring.[45] Put another way, their absence can well be destabilizing to the client and her situation.**

The agency's presence, *qua* presence, should also be viewed as a stabilizing force. It is a visible source of involvement and hope to the client and the community. In the best situations it is a "positive disruption" of a pathological process or way of life.

---

*Along with Butler and Lewis we would agree that "When in doubt, treat. . ." A central premise of this article and the work herein described is that one starts the work before all the facts are in.

**In a few instances it is recognized that some people would be better off "out," either for their own or your client's mental health. Even then one moves cautiously. The point of examination being the "cost" of being out, to the client, to the person, and to the agency.

Linkages

The third dimension, linkage, completes the treatment structure. In practice, stabilization and linkage often occur together, the latter providing the former. No one agency can do everything. One sensible approach is to work cooperatively with other organizations that are best at their specific tasks. The total service package needed is then delivered, and at a good quality level. The linkages may be to formal organizations such as a Social Security Office, to volunteer groups as found in churches, or to neighbors.

Mr. M.'s friend, who did the shopping needed to be away for a few weeks. Mr. M. was wheelchair bound and fearful of leaving his apartment. The agency helped secure SSI by having them make a home visit (Mr. M. was unable to make this request himself of SSI, though once engaged in the face-to-face, he was assertive). Large print books were provided. A church provided twice a week "friendly visitors" (their term) as part of their ministry. The volunteers were supposed to read to Mr. M., but he was so enthusiastic for an audience and so full of stories that the volunteers often brought a friend who listened to a time past. (His having been in the Foreign Legion, been a part of the "Old West," and a world traveler, all made him a romantic figure.) Later in consultation with his friend, Meals on Wheels provided lunches.

Several things were notable. Each linkage was dual; i.e., directed to and from the agency, as well as to Mr. M. Several were somewhat official in their construction, viz., securing SSI and a home attendant. The "friendly visitors," the Meals on Wheels, and the library came because they were asked to by the agency. Their relationships with the agency were such that the referral was "trusted." They also knew that the agency was there to assist and advise them as the need arose. Mr. M. would and could not be their burden alone. It seems that services are provided not only on the basis of need (a clear ideological dimension), but such provision is enhanced by an agency maintaining excellent relations with other members of a service network.

The provision of a home attendant is of great importance. The exact duties to be performed need to be carefully laid out, again with the guiding notion of supplementing, not supplanting, what other caregivers do. It is also advantageous to provide ongoing support and supervision for them. The office is the preferred locale, and, if possible, attendants should be paid for their time. In these ways the home attendant can feel that her contributions, insights, and work, are important. Persons involved in such situations need to feel that they are not working in isolation, that they are part of a team.[46]

The above example is devoid of an important group of services, viz., medical. Mr. M. refused to leave his apartment and hadn't seen a physician in years. More pathologically, he refused to let a doctor visit him, though such was available. (Three exams were in order: a general physical; a psychiatric evaluation; and, an opthamological one.) The reasons for refusal were clear, and seemingly unshakeable. His last exam had resulted in a second amputation and a brief nursing home placement. Establishing this critical linkage became an important goal. The agency "eased" its way toward it by having the nurse visit him.

Why did the linkages take the shape they did? As noted, Mr. M. was a full participant in defining what the service package would look like. (With less alert clients the agency, independently of the client, may well have to define the needs, as well as set up, and monitor the service system.) His definition was not wholly consistent with the agency's in priority or structure. In the latter instance the agency thought that the library program was superfluous as he became less and less able to read; he thought otherwise, wanting the company of both the books and their deliverer. The dual priorities of getting him outside the apartment and examined medically were regarded as being of little consequence by him.

This example also suggests the range of linkages that are possible. Some clients will need (or accept) less, others more. The totality looks different in each situation. The worker maximizes her skill and the benefit given, by linking up the needed resources. Knowledge and respect for all parts of the team is a *sine qua non.*

The hard work in setting up a good and helpful linkage system,* the calling to attention of gaps in service and trying to fill them, neither obviates the need, nor excuses the agency from providing an ongoing therapeutic relationship.

---

*Where reimbursement is only for face-to-face interviews, the cost of setting up a linkage system is formidable. No real solution is here offered beyond noting that, for this client group, linkages are crucial to continued mental health, and agencies must strive to have this recognized and accepted.

Process

The triad of beginnings, stabilization, and linkage, define major portions of a strategy of intervention with the mentally frail elderly. Social work's work, at base, is process oriented. The social worker's actions and behaviors are as much goal oriented, as directed towards the establishment and maintenance of a particular process. The underpinning of the process is the relationship between the worker and the client.[47] For the mentally frail elderly this relationship may extend through a client's lifetime. The agency must be prepared, and expect, to make such a commitment.

> Mr. C. rarely kept appointments; his attendance in a group had been equally sporadic over several years. When he did come in, he expressed a clear desire and need for therapy. To the group he generally explained his irregularity as "just wanting to say hello" or to celebrate a holiday together with them.

Mr. C. was a cipher, each reappearance a new, yet familiar beginning. The staff felt a sense of failure for not "really" engaging him. He seemed to know, better than any one when to come. Returns to the agency, and its continuing acceptance provided sustenance, strength and identification. It may be argued that Mr. C. had a great number of problems on which work needed to be done and was not. This is accurate. The agency must stand ready, when and if the time comes, for ongoing work.

Simultaneously, it provides what services it can. Thus, when a medical emergency arose and Mr. C. was hospitalized, he asked the agency to maintain his affairs. His social security check was entrusted to the social worker to pay rent and other bills. He signed a "power of attorney" so that his wishes would be carried out should he be unable to do so. The worker and group members visited, reciprocating his attention to them.

With their informed participation and consent an agency may handle the affairs of clients. Protection of living space, payment of utilities, purchasing food, arranging for a phone, shopping for clothing (together, when possible), etc., are all important tasks. Performing these activities, as part of a treatment plan, reduces stress. Equally important, they are intrinsic parts of the process. Thus, all activities become legitimate objects of explanation, examination, and evaluation between the worker and client.

Workers must constantly test the limits of comprehension with the mentally frail elderly.

> Miss B. was severely organic. Little seemed to stimulate her, though she liked to sit by the window of her hotel room. Her worker one day suggested that she might enjoy the company of others, as in a nursing home. Miss B. replied, "No. I want to finish by sitting and looking at my Broadway."

This was the first full and truly coherent statement Miss B. had made in a year. Her grasp of her situation was striking, and accurate. The work supports and expands upon the presented strengths, internal as well as external.

Where a client is realistically unable to participate, the agency may have to seek protective services.[48] Each agency must examine the extent to which it can be the provider of such service. Their presence or absence does not, and should not, preclude the agency from being the provider of social work and mental health services, any more than the presence or absence of any other service would. The social worker through knowing the many connected parts of a situation and by virtue of her knowledge of process can look upon herself as being the central person (aside from the client) in a case, though not necessarily the most important at any given moment.

Goals

For each case specific goals are made, individualizing each client. However, a general perspective is possible. Each worker articulates their agency's purpose in setting broad goals of a case. The translation from philosophy to practice and purpose is an ongoing task. Thus, such notions as preventing or delaying institutionalization, improving interpersonal relationships, minimizing stress, and the like are at once unique and general. Some examples will clarify this.

One general goal is to take a walk with your client, trying to see the world from her perspective, from her pace. This serves diagnostic functions, is enjoyable, and can be a genuine sharing.

> Ms. N. was articulate, publicly joyful and incontinent. One day her worker returning to the office from the field, saw her walking and asked to join her. Ms. N. told her that it had been

years since anyone had walked with her. She also pointed out many people previously available only in descriptions, and even proudly introduced the worker to several. For the first time Ms. N. admitted her loneliness and frustration, of the isolating consequences of her condition, though the worker had long believed this to be the case. Prior to "the walk" she had denied such. The worker often met her afterwards and they walked together, the walk sometimes becoming the session.

A second general goal of a community-based service is to have the client come to the office. Many situations must start in the home, the worker having to make home visits in order to engage the client, or the client being physically unable to travel. However, the home is not therapeutically neutral.

> 'I'm not so glad you came today,' Mrs. V. told the worker. 'The CIA has been watching me through the TV again. I better not say anything more.'

The office isn't really neutral either. It should be a therapeutically positive place and space. One of the ways the ongoing process differs from beginnings is that the worker strives to make the healthy familiar and acceptable. The client then may be perceived of as being ready to "go to the healthy," not just have it come to her.

The delusional pattern of Mrs. V. is hard to break. Office visits may be encouraged by initially making such a visit social ("I really would like you to see where I work."), or even a ceremonial occasion. ("I'd like you to meet my boss.") This helps the client to identify with the agency; demonstrates that the worker is not ashamed to be seen with the client; and, that the worker wants to share an important aspect of their life with the client. The worker should introduce the client to whoever is available. Visits should be planned when the executive will be available. People not only deserve, but respond to, respect.[49]

Another general goal is to maximize usage of available resources, as seen in the example of Mr. M. Benefits as rights (justice), rather than charity, is a cornerstone of such explanation and negotiation.[50]

It is almost redundant to speak of building upon a client's strengths, Yet, faced with overwhelming pathology and tragedy, one can forget this. Clients will remind us of its essential truth.

Mrs. Z. an 80 year old with emphysema had known much better times socially, emotionally, and financially. Diagnosed as a paranoid schizophrenic, she seemed to work at living up to most of its clinical manifestations. Nursing students were hesitantly sent in to monitor her physical signs. It was like a scene from a movie where the wise old patient instructs the scared intern. Mrs. Z. never tired, until her death some years later, of teaching.

The Z case brings forth a dual message. First, that critical goals are to help give a person a sense of worth, of participation in life about them.[51] Second, that there is work for each person to do. There is the internal psychic work which a social worker psychotherapist can help guide; and, there is the external work, the societal participative work that brings wholeness.[52] Mrs. Z. received deep gratification that she still had a useful role in life.

This work, like all work, is bound by the limited time available. The wounds and the reality run very deep and are difficult to fully counter or change. Sights need to be set towards the possible. This leads to a notion of "good time." One works to create such a period, for however long it may last. With Ms. D., described earlier, the "good time" lasted nearly two years. With her worker's assistance she started coming out during the day, dressed appropriately, allowed repairs to her room, went to a center, and reestablished a relationship with a grand nephew, her only surviving relative. The etiology of the deterioration was probably several subacute strokes and her grand nephew's moving some distance away. It became time to renew the interventive process, the "good time" was drawing to an end. Ms. D's. success was an important diagnostic tool and source of strength for rebuilding.

There has been some attention given to reminiscence of late.[53] It is important that the worker listen to the client's life. The sense of passing something of themselves on, as in the case of Mr. M., is an important part of the work. Process and goal intermingle to form a whole in this activity.

SUMMING UP

A triad of causes is noted for the etiology of an emerging and visible group of the mentally frail and disabled elderly, the permanent patient. This appellation conveys a status and condition quite accurately. Such usage also helps sensitize agencies and workers to the extent of case need and longevity. Psychiatric involvement with the elderly, except diagnostically, has been minimal. Social work skills and services should be the primary locus for emphasis and training. A model of service in which the intervention is conceptualized as consisting of beginnings, stabilization, and linkage is outlined. These three overlapping dimensions clarify stages of the process, allowing a worker and her agency to work with, as well as for, the permanent patient.

Finally, we see that case activities, and the strategies of intervention outlined, are directed towards two overlapping goals. First, to provide life-sustaining needs, such as housing, food, medical care, and clothing. Second, to reestablish the social order, i.e., to provide normative expectations to the greatest possible degree. These expectations flow as much towards the client, as from her. They also flow within, closing a circle of interaction; one in which participation, as an essential of all human life, is reconstituted.

REFERENCES

1. Anderson, Odin. "Reflections on the Sick Aged and the Helping Systems." *Social Policy, Social Ethics, and the Aging Society*. Edited by Bernice Neugarten and Robert Havighurst. Washington, D.C.: National Science Foundation, 1976.

Dobrof, Rose and Litwak, Eugene. *Maintenance of Family Ties of Long-Term Care Patients: Theory and Guide to Practice*. Washington, D.C.: H.E.W., 1977.

Frolich, Philip. *The 1967 National Survey of Institutionalized Adults: Residents Long-Term Medical Care Institutions*. Washington, D.C.: H.E.W., 1974.

Kane, Rosalie and Kane, Robert. *Assessing the Elderly: A Practical Guide to Measurement*. Lexington, Mass.: Lexington Books, 1981.

Laird, Carobeth. *Limbo*. Novato, Ca.: Chandler & Sharp, 1979.

Smith, David. *Long Term Care in Transition: The Regulation of Nursing Homes*. Washington, D.C.: AUPHA Press, 1981.

Thomas, William. *Nursing Homes and Public Policy: Drift and Decision in New York State*. Ithaca: Cornell University Press, 1969.

U.S. Congress: Special Committee on Aging, U.S. Senate—Subcommittee on Long Term Care. *Nursing Home Care in the U.S.: Failure in Public Policy*. (7 vols.) Washington, D.C.; G.P.O., 1974-76.

Vladeck, Bruce. *Unloving Care: The Nursing Home Tragedy*. New York: Basic Books.

2. Kane, Robert and Kane, Rosalie. "Care of the Aged: Old Problems in Need of New Solutions," *Science* 200 (26 May 1978), 913-919.

Berezin, Martin. "Psychodynamic Considerations of Aging and the Aged: An Overview," *American Journal of Psychiatry*, 128 (June 1972), 33-41.

3. Baxter, Ellen and Hopper, Kim. *Private Lives/Public Spaces: Homeless Adults on the Streets of New York City*. New York: Community Service Society, 1981.

Rousseau, Ann. *Shopping Bag Ladies*. New York: Pilgrim Press, 1981.

4. President's Commission on Mental Health. *Report to the President*. Washington,

D.C.: The Commission, 1978 (4 volumes). See esp. Vol. 1, *Mental Health in America, 1978.*

5. Tourney, Garfield. "Psychiatric Therapies: 1880-1968," *Changing Patterns in Psychiatric Care.* Edited by Theodore Rothman. New York: Crown, 1970.

6. Caudill, William. *The Psychiatric Hospital as a Small Society.* Cambridge, Ma.: Harvard, 1958.

Stanton, Alfred and Schwartz, Morris. *The Mental Hospital: A Study of Institutional Participation on Psychiatric Illness and Treatment.* New York: Basic Books, 1954.

7. Caudill. *Ibid.*

Goffman, Erving. *Asylums.* New York: Doubleday, 1961.

8. Blatt, Burton. *Souls in Extremis.* Boston: Allyn and Bacon, 1973.

Greenblatt, Milton. "The Evolution of State Mental Hospital Models of Treatment." *Further Explorations in Social Psychiatry.* Edited by Berton Kaplan, Robert Wilson, and Alexander Leighton. New York: Basic Books, 1976.

Laird. *Ibid.*

9. Beigel, Allan and Levenson, Alan. "The Community Mental Health Center: Origin and Concepts." *The Community Mental Health Center.* Edited by Allan Biegel and Alan Levenson. New York: Basic Books, 1972.

The *Community Mental Health Centers Act of 1963.* P.L. 88-164.

Olander, Helen. "Health Services: Community Mental Health." *Encyclopedia of Social Work,* 17th Edition. Washington, D.C.: NASW, 1977.

10. Moroney, Robert. *Families, Social Services and Social Policy: The Issue of Shared Responsibility.* Washington, D.C.: N.I.M.H. 1980. The rates per 1,000 of elderly in mental hospitals dropped from 4.07 in 1950 to 2.13 in 1970 (Table 14).

The 1955 New York State Hospital population was 93,337. By mid-1980 it was 24,581. cf. New York City Department of Mental Health, *Mental Health Plan for Homeless Adults in New York City,* 1981.

11. Kane, Robert and Kane, Rosalie. *Ibid.*

Maddox, George. "The Continuum of Care: Movement Toward the Community." *Handbook of Geriatric Psychiatry.* Edited by Ewald Busse and Dan Blazer. New York: Van Nostrand, 1980.

Moroney. *Ibid.* The Rate of institutionalized elderly in Nursing Homes and Homes for the Aged rose from 1.96 to 4.56 per 1,000 between 1950 and 1970 (Table 14).

12. Gurian, Bennett. "Mental Health and the Aging." *Improving the Quality of Health Care for the Elderly.* Edited by John Brookbank. Gainesville, Fla.: University Presses, 1978.

13. Cummings, John and Cummings, Elaine. "Care in the Community," *Modern Perspectives in the Psychiatry of Old Age.* Edited by John Howells. New York: Brunner/Mazel, 1975.

14. New York State, *Mental Hygiene Law,* Article 9.

15. Laird. *Ibid.*

Mendelson, Mary. *Tender Loving Greed.* New York: Random House, 1974.

Townsend, Claire. *Old Age: The Last Segregation.* New York: Grossman, 1971.

16. Neugarten, Bernice. "Age Groups in American Society and the Rise of the Young-Old," *The Annals,* 415 (Sept. 1974).

17. Federal Council on Aging. *The Need for Long-Term Care.* Washington, D.C.: H.H.S., 1981. (Esp. Charts 1.1 & 1.2).

18. Lawton, M. Powell and Hoover, Sally, Eds. *Community Housing Choices for Older Americans.* New York: Springer, 1981 (Esp. Chapters 1-4).

New York Times. 12/1/81; 12/5/81; 12/28/81; 1/15/82, etc. The impact, and reports of it, are frequent.

19. Gurian. *Ibid.*

20. ". . . as we wish our own. . . " is a positive stereotype. Deviations from this provide a useful, though inexact, definitional structure.

21. Becker, Howard. *Outsiders.* New York: The Free Press, 1963.

Goffman, Erving. *Stigma: Notes on the Management of Spoiled Identity.* Englewood Cliffs: Prentice Hall, 1963.

David Feldstein   139

22. Ryan, William. *Blaming the Victim, Revised Ed.* New York: Random House (Vintage Books), 1976.
23. Hochchild, Arlie. *The Unexpected Community: Portrait of an Old Age Subculture.* Berkeley: University of California Press, 1973.
24. Cummings & Cummings. *Ibid.*
25. Goffman. *Stigma,* Op. Cit.
26. Baxter & Hopper. *Ibid.*
The City of New York, President of the City Council. *From County Asylums to City Streets: The Contradiction Between Deinstitutionalization and State Mental Health Funding Priorities.* ("The Bellamy Report"), 1979.
Rousseau. *Ibid.*
Young, Randy. "The Homeless: The Shame of the City," *New York* 14, 21 December 1981, (26-32).
27. Federal Council on Aging, *Ibid* (Charts 1.1, 1.5, 1.7-1.12).
28. Des Pres, Terrence. *The Survivor.* New York: Oxford University Press, 1976 (See esp. pp. 23-26).
29. Quoted by Lazarus, Lawrence and Weinberg, Jack. "Treatment in the Ambulatory Care Setting." *Handbook. . .* Edited by Busse and Blazer, *Op. Cit.*
30. Quoted in Kane, Robert et al. "The Future Need for Geriatric Manpower in the United States," *New England Journal of Medicine* 302 (12 June 1980), 1327-1332.
Redich, Richard; Kramer, Morton; and Taube, Carl. "Epidemiology of Mental Illness and Utilization of Psychiatric Facilities Among Older Persons." *Mental Illness in Later Life.* Edited by Ewald Busse and Eric Pfeiffer. Washington, D.C.: American Psychiatric Association, 1973.
31. Robinson, R.A. "The Assessment Center." *Modern Perspectives . . .* Ed. by John Howells, *Op. Cit.*
32. Private communications with members of the Group for Geriatric Psychiatry of New York.
33. American Psychiatric Association. *Diagnostic and Statistical Manual of Mental Disorders, 3rd Edition* (DSM-111). Washington, D.C.: A.P.A., 1980.
34. Hollis, Florence. *Casework: A Psychosocial Therapy, 2nd Edition.* New York: Random House, 1972 (Esp. Chapters 7, 10, 14-17).
Perlman, Helen. *Social Casework: A Problem Solving Process.* Chicago: The University Press, 1957 (esp. Chapters 1-7 and 11).
Reid, William and Epstein, Laura. *Task-Centered Casework.* New York: Columbia University Press, 1972 (Esp. Chapters 1 & 3).
35. Lazarus and Weinberg, *Op. Cit.,* p. 431.
36. Giannturco, Daniel and Busse, Ewald. "Psychiatric Problems Encountered During a Long Term Study of Normal Aging Volunteers." *Studies in Geriatric Psychiatry.* Edited by Anthony Isaacs and Felix Post. New York: John Wiley and Sons, 1978.
37. Butler, Robert. "Aging: Research Leads and Needs," *Forum on Medicine* 2, 11/79 (716-725).
38. Butler, Robert and Lewis, Myrna. *Aging and Mental Health.* St. Louis: C.V. Mosby, 1973 (Esp. pp. 143-185).
Giannturco & Busse. *Ibid.*
Marsden, C.D. "The Diagnosis of Dementia." *Studies in . . .* Ed. by Isaacs & Post, *Op. Cit.*
Voerward, Adrian. *Clinical Geropsychiatry.* Baltimore: Williams and Wilkens, 1976 (Esp. pp. 11-131).
Wang, H. Shan. "Special Diagnostic Procedures—The Evaluation of Brain Impairment," *Mental Illness. . .* Edited by Busse and Pfeiffer, *op. cit.*
39. Marsden, *Ibid,* p. 116.
40. Riffer, N. et al. *Case Management Services in Community Support Systems—A Training Manual.* New York and Albany: New York State Office of Mental Health, N.D.
Rosenthal, Stephen and Levine, Edith. "Case Management and Policy Implementation," *Public Policy,* 28 (Fall 1980), 381-413.

41. Butler & Lewis, *Ibid*, p. 139.
42. Gurian, *Ibid*, p. 70.
43. Goldfarb, Alvin and Turner, Helen. "Psychotherapy of Aged Persons: Utilization and Effectiveness of 'Brief' Therapy," *American Journal of Psychiatry*, 109 (1953), 916-921.
44. Hollis. *Ibid.*
   Perlman. *Ibid.*
   Reid and Epstein. *Ibid.*
   Richmond, Mary. *Social Diagnosis.* New York: Russell Sage, 1917.
45. Dobrof & Litwak. *Ibid.*
   Moroney. *Ibid.*
46. Schwartz, Florence. Personal Communication.
47. Germain, Carel and Gitterman, Alex. *The Life Model of Social Work Practice.* New York: Columbia, 1980.
   Hollis. *Ibid.*
   Perlman. *Ibid.*
   Reid. *Ibid.*
48. Schoenfeld, Barbara and Tuzil, Teresa. "Conservatorship: A Move Towards More Personalized Protective Service," *Journal of Gerontological Social Work*, 1 (Spring, 1979), 225-234.
   United States Senate, Special Committee on Aging. *Protective Services for the Elderly.* Washington, D.C.: Special Committee, 1977.
49. Towle, Charlotte. *Common Human Needs*, rev. ed. New York: NASW, 1957.
50. Also, Note F. supra.
   Rawls, John. *A Theory of Justice.* Cambridge, Ma.: Harvard U. Press, 1971 (Esp. Ch. 1 & 11, part 16).
51. Zaborowski, Mark and Herzog, Elizabeth. *Life is With People.* New York: Schocken, 1962.
52. Butler & Lewis, *Ibid.*
   Erikson, Erik. *Childhood and Society.* New York: Norton, 1950 (Esp. Ch. 7).
53. Lesser, Jory et al. "Reminiscence Group Therapy with Psychotic Geriatric In-patients," *The Gerontologist* 21 (June 1981), 291-296.
   Lewis, Myrna and Butler, Robert. "Life Review Therapy: Putting Memories of Work in Individual and Group Psychotherapy," *Geriatrics* 29 (November 1974), 165-174.
   Merriam, Sharon. "The Concept and function of Reminiscence: A Review of the Research," *The Gerontologist* 20 (October 1980), 604-609.

Chapter IX

Emotional Stresses in Later Life

Harriet Rzetelny

For a year you mourn, and after that you have to go on
with your life, that's the Law
The rabbi told me: If you go on crying and mourning,
there is no peace, the year is up.

The year is never up.
This morning I was going to bake some potatoes and
my sister came back to me, how she used to brush the
potatoes.
It never stops.

Hilda Glick, Bella Jacobskind, Vera Rosenfeld[1*]

If any stress can be particularly associated with old age it is the
stress resulting from loss. People of all ages experience loss. Aside
from the obvious losses such as death of parents, early widowhood
and economic failure, people experience a sense of loss as they give
up one life stage to move into another as, for example, when they
lose the freedom of young adulthood to marry and raise a family.
The majority of people who suffer early and mid-life losses can find
replacements: remarriage, starting again in business, finding new
friends, etc. Gradually the effects of the losses are lessened as people move on and reinvest their emotional energy into new ventures
and new people.
People in late life suffer many losses, often within a short period
of time, and they suffer these losses at a stage in life when physiological reserve and opportunities for replacement, substitution and

---

*The poems used in the text were written by the members of the JASA Brooklyn Poetry
Clubs and quoted by Marc Kaminsky in his book on working with older people: *What's Inside You. It Shines Out Of You.* New York: Horizon Press, 1974.

141

gratification are at their lowest. In contemporary western society, entering the last stage of life offers little compensation for having lost the authority, status and financial control of the middle years. Few opportunities exist for older people to pass on their accumulated knowledge and experience in any meaningful way. Ego integration[2]—that which Erikson defines as the last task of identity formation—often takes place in the midst of crippling poverty and deplorable living conditions while younger people hurry by uncaring and unseeing. The struggle for survival in a nonsupportive environment can substantiate older people's worst fears about themselves. It can seem as though sickness, frailty, loss and poverty are just deserts for not planning better, not working harder, or not being a "better" person.

The losses of later life can be broken roughly into four categories:

1. *The Aging Process.* The losses resulting from the physiological aging processes such as psychomotor impairment and joint degeneration, sensory loss and loss of physiological reserve. Although these losses are gradual and take place over time, allowing most people to make the necessary adjustments and adaptations, they make coping with other losses that much more difficult.

2. *Health.* The loss of health which can occur suddenly as with a stroke, or gradually as with a chronic condition such as emphysema. Illness, especially where the resulting incapacitation lasts a long time or is permanent, can be devastating to an older person, in part because of the potential it has for triggering other losses such as loss of independence, loss of mobility and loss of opportunities for social, vocational and avocational activities.

The advent of a serious illness is often the first time that older people must struggle with the realities of the aging processes which slow down recovery, and must confront their own mortality. Acute anxiety frequently accompanies even minor illnesses, especially in situations where a frail older person may already be coping at the limits of her emotional and physical capacity. At this point, any additional stress can upset the fragile balance she may be maintaining between her inner resources and the demands of reality, and a minor illness can be perceived as a major threat.[3]

3. *Death of Others.* Death of significant people who comprise the emotional support system of an older person such as spouse, siblings and friends. The importance of significant relationships in the lives

of older people cannot be overemphasized. For a vulnerable, impaired older person, the presence of one person who can offer emotional support and assistance with vital activities of daily life can make the difference between the ability to remain in the community or the necessity for institutionalization.

4. *The social and environmental losses* of aging such as loss of income, status, meaningful and productive social roles and activities, and the possible resultant loss of respect and self-esteem.

GRIEF AND MOURNING

Grief and mourning are a natural and necessary response to any loss, not just death. Grief can be defined as the emotional reaction to a loss; the feelings of shock, anger, betrayal, helplessness, hopelessness, sadness, etc. Mourning is the process by which grief is resolved, the loss is gradually accepted, and the individual becomes free to invest emotional energy into something or someone else. This process can take varying amounts of time depending on the extent and significance of the loss, and the emotional ability of the person to actively and openly engage in grief work. The normal range is between six and eighteen months.[4]

Until he suffered a stroke, Mr. Reynolds, age 78, had been functioning fairly well despite some arthritis and a partial cataract. Always a proud and independent man, he maintained his own apartment with some assistance from his daughter who shopped for him when the weather prohibited his going out. He attended a local senior citizen's club to play cards with his friends two or three times a week.

Following his stroke he had a brief stay in a convalescent home where he regained almost full mobility and speech, although his left side remained slightly paralyzed. Upon his return home he sat himself in front of the television set and refused to budge despite entreaties from his daughter and the worker employed by the senior citizen's club who visited him in his home. "I'm a useless old man," he'd say bitterly. "Don't bother with me. My body is no good anymore. Just let me sit here." "Don't say that," his daughter would answer. "There's nothing wrong with you." Her father would turn away without answering, but would explode with rage if she was late for a visit or bought him the wrong brand of pipe tobacco.

The center worker was able to help Mr. Reynolds' daughter understand that in addition to his anxieties regarding his own survival, her father was grieving for the loss of his body image and body function. Although most of his mobility had returned, Mr. Reynolds had not yet completed his grief work. He felt betrayed and abandoned by a body that had given out on him, leaving him helpless and paralyzed. Angry at his loss of independence, with his ability to master his environment impaired, he struck out at his daughter whose independence and mobility was intact. With increased understanding, Mr. Reynold's daughter was able to help her father verbalize some of his feelings and understand that they were natural and normal. Together with the center worker, she was able to help him accept his loss and his limitations and become reinvolved with his life and his friends.

I sat on the family plot. There was my father, there was my mother, there was my brother, there was my sister, and I was the only alive person here.

Hilda Glick, Bella Jacobskind, Vera Rosenfeld[1]

DEPRESSION

For many older people, loss follows loss and grief work is never completed. Underlying, unresolved feelings, often too overwhelming and complex to be articulated, can crystallize into depression. Depression is by far the most common emotional problem of late life. Some people have grown old with depression. They may have lived their lives with an ongoing, underlying depression erupting into periods of acute, depressive episodes effecting work, education and/or relationships. The losses and increased vulnerability of old age can trigger or intensify such a preexisting condition. It is very difficult for workers without special training to treat this kind of depression.

Many other people experience acute or reactive depression for the first time in old age. A reactive depression can be thought of as grief and mourning turned inward. It is also triggered by a loss, frequently by a series of losses but unlike normal grief, the individual is usually unaware of the connection between the losses and the feelings being experienced. The feelings themselves are often blurred and blunted and the person feels heavy, despondent or angry without knowing why. Workers should be aware that the symptoms of depression occur in many disguised forms. Depression is frequently expressed in the form of physical complaints. Problems with digestion and elimination, sudden weight loss or weight gain, early morning wakefulness, inability to sleep or chronic fatigue can all be symptoms of depression.[5]

Mrs. Turner, age 74, became a widow thirteen months ago. She had always taken an interest in community affairs and, following a brief mourning period, she became involved in her community recreation program as a volunteer. High blood pressure and shortness of breath made it difficult for her to work, but it wasn't until she suffered a mild heart attack that her doctor insisted that she give up her volunteer job. Subsequently, Mrs. Turner began complaining of difficulty falling asleep accompanied by daily fatigue. Always a hearty eater, Mrs. Turner began to feel that certain foods were not agreeing with her and soon lost fifteen pounds. "I don't know what's wrong with me," she said to concerned friends. "I simply don't feel like myself."

Mrs. Turner did not connect her physical and emotional state with the loss of her volunteer job following upon her heart attack and the loss of her husband. Mrs. Turner's doctor diagnosed a reactive depression. After he helped her to discuss her feelings of anger and despondency at her losses and to understand what was happening to her, Mrs. Turner became involved as a volunteer with a telephone reassurance program. This did not require as much physical exertion as did her former job. Within a short time, her appetite and sleep problems disappeared.

Alcohol abuse, when it begins or intensifies late in life, can also signify depression. Typically, the individual is never seen drinking but an alert worker can note some of the signals: alcohol on the breath when the older person arrives at the recreation or lunch program; unexplained bruises and discolorations from falls; time lapses, especially in the evenings and on weekends, when the older person appears vague or confused about what she has done or where she has been but is not otherwise confused or disoriented; a general impression of loneliness, isolation or lack of any meaningful activities or relationships outside of the particular program the individual attends.

Alcohol abuse in the form of solitary drinking becomes more difficult to treat the longer it has been established as a way of life and a way of numbing or suppressing feelings. Caught early and dealt with as a symptom of depression, the older person can be helped to establish new interests and activities as a replacement for the drinking.[6]

> There will come a day
> When you won't remember what happened yesterday
> You go to the drawer
> & you don't remember what you came for.
>
> My daughter—I hate to tell her the bad.
> But to you: I can tell this.
>
> Beatrice Zucker, Hilda Glick, Marc Kaminsky[1]

Depression in late life can also look like some of the early symptoms of senile dementia.* Memory loss can serve as a protective device for an older person to whom the realities of life are painful. There is a fine but important distinction between "I can't remember" and "I don't want to remember because remembering will make me sad or anxious." Depression can also be an emotional reaction to the beginnings of an organic condition. It is important that workers be aware that depression and senile dementia so often go hand in hand. A person in the early stages of dementia can be helped to mourn the loss of his mental abilities and to continue with life to the extent of his capacities.

Although both depression and dementia may be present, the following may help the worker distinguish between the two. People in the beginning stages of an organic impairment tend to want to conceal their disabilities. When asked a question that involves reasoning ability or arithmetic, they will guess at the answer. Occasionally they are right, but more often they are wrong. A depressed person is more likely to say "I don't know. My mind is no

---

*The following discussion and case example are adapted from an earlier chapter which appeared in Working with Frail Elderly in Senior Centers by Harriet Rzetelny. Brookdale Center on Aging of Hunter College and NYS Department of Social Services, 1981.

good anymore.'' Depressed people need to communicate the way they feel about themselves, their helplessness, hopelessness and sadness. People feeling the shame and humiliation of declining mental abilities are more likely to try to hide it.

Another clue is to observe what the older person remembers and when he remembers it. If he doesn't remember the name of the state his daughter moved to or the name of the man he worked for, but remembers all other names, his memory failure may be related more to the losses involved than to an organic impairment. If he doesn't remember where he put things when he is home alone but remembers them when he is with others, his memory failure may be related to loneliness.[7]

> Mr. Matthews is a seventy-year old retired factory foreman who moved to the town where his daughter was living five years ago in order to live with her. Nine months ago his daughter died. He stayed on in the apartment by himself, taking his major meal at a local senior center. The center worker wanted him to participate in some of the other activities such as the current events club. His response was, 'My mind is too old. The last president I remember is Nixon whose daughter married what's his name's son. See, I can't even remember who she married. After Nixon, they're all blurry to me.'

> The worker then suggested that he join the carpentry group as this was an activity he enjoyed when he was younger. To this his response was, 'Carpentry? To do carpentry you have to be able to read the blueprints. When I was the foreman I could read the blueprints. Now I can't read the blueprints anymore. They're just a bunch of lines. My mind is getting worse every day.'[11]

There is no way of knowing for sure whether or not Mr. Matthews has the beginnings of an organic condition, but he is suffering from depression. He remembers Nixon's daughter but can't remember who she married, a clue that he is still dealing with the loss of his daughter. His inability to read the blueprints appears to be a selective mental problem; more an indication of his feelings of uselessness and reduced self-esteem, and he is managing to pay his bills and maintain his apartment which he would have difficulty doing without assistance if he was suffering from an organic impairment. Mr. Matthews is not attempting to cover his memory loss. Rather, he is using his condition as a way of communicating his emotional state.

PARANOIA

Another reaction to emotional stress in older people is paranoia. Loneliness, isolation, reduced hearing and vision, anxiety over failing mental and physical abilities may result in a paranoid episode or a simple delusion. A delusion is defined as "a firm, fixed idea not amenable to rational explanation, maintained despite logical argument and objective, contradictory evidence."[8]

It may be less anxiety producing to an older person to believe that someone stole his social security check rather than to admit to himself that he can't remember where he put it. A vulnerable older person struggling to survive with failing eyesight or hearing can easily feel threatened and misconstrue what people say or what he thinks he sees.

People who evidence paranoia in late life were probably somewhat mistrustful and suspicious as younger people. They may have found it difficult to establish new relationships when a trusted spouse or sibling died. Paranoid people seek confirmation of their worst fears in order to justify them. They need to believe that the source of their anxiety is located in the outside world and does not come from within them. Attempts to prove to paranoid older people that their delusions are groundless will only heighten their inner anxiety, and this they cannot tolerate. As a defense, they will maintain an even greater belief in their delusion.

The clue to working with a paranoid older person is to help reduce their inner anxiety. Establish yourself as a person they can trust by being completely trustworthy. Never promise anything you can't deliver. Never lie to a paranoid person, because lying or even simple evasion of the truth is like waving a red flag in front of a bull and will destroy any trust that might ever have developed. Providing concrete services to enhance security, or a hearing aid to better interpret environmental clues may prove more fruitful.

SUPPORT SYSTEMS OF THE FRAIL ELDERLY

The importance of a reliable, dependable "other" in the life of a frail older person cannot be too strongly emphasized. As spouse, family or peer group die or move away, community workers who are in regular, ongoing contact with older people take on a special significance in their lives. They often provide the emotional lifeline essential to a vulnerable older person struggling to survive.

Older people do not use services designated as "mental health services" in any appreciable numbers; partly because these services are not readily available for older people and partly because of the stigma attached to using such services. Any community service such as a nutrition or recreation program, a senior center, homecare or escort service becomes, in effect, a mental health service because such services support older people's coping efforts and help them in their struggle to maintain their independence and dignity. Older people, in return, invest emotion and meaning into their relationship with the workers in these programs, often far beyond the parameters of the service or to a degree beyond which the worker may expect or feel comfortable in receiving.

When older people do have surviving children, the familial relationships may be ambivalent or stressful, as children and their parents struggle to adjust to changing needs, expectations and roles. Older people are very sensitive about being burdens to their children. Children may become irrationally angry at their parents for not remaining the strong, reliable symbol of home and security they once were. The worker-client relationship, on the other hand, can be one of the few relatively conflict-free significant relationships in older people's lives. It can provide older people with the opportunity to sort through their feelings, mourn their losses and create order and meaning from their experiences by reminiscing, story telling, or just plain sharing the past with someone who is an outsider yet can listen and respond with sensitivity.

Community workers do not have to enter into traditional counseling relationships with older people in order to help them in this way. A bus trip, a wait in the clinic or Medicaid center, a few minutes in the worker's office or the client's home over a cup of tea can provide the opportunity for a word of understanding.

THE SOCIAL WORK ROLE

Briefly described below are some of the ways that a sensitive worker can help an older person to cope with late-life stresses.

  a. *Legitimize feelings*. Older people need to know that their feelings are understandable and acceptable, especially their angry or negative feelings. Workers who are not afraid of their own feelings can help an older person to understand that it is natural to be angry at a dying spouse or a friend who moved away and left them.

b. *Absolve from guilt.* As people sort through their lives, self-serving acts or deeds left undone can be sources of unresolved guilt. Older people often have unrealistic expectations of themselves. A woman caring for a disabled spouse, for example, may feel guilty if she spends time away from her husband's side. She needs reassurance that time away for herself is absolutely necessary if she is to continue to provide emotional sustenance to her husband. An understanding word from a trusted and respected worker can help an older person struggling to put his life into order to feel that he's done the best he can.

c. *Support coping efforts.* Older people may feel hopeless and overwhelmed when loss follows loss and they do not overcome the loss as quickly as they once did. A worker can help by pointing out how they have coped with losses or problems in the past. The fact that a woman has survived into her 80's means that she has good survival skills, a fact that is often forgotten by older people and the people who work with them.

d. *Support autonomy and decision making.* A sense of mastery or control over one's environment is essential for good self-esteem and healthy functioning. Older people will often "trade in" their decision making perogatives if that is the only way they can obtain the help and assistance that they need. But the capitulation is frequently a painful one, fraught with hidden resentments, self-blame and feelings of degredation. Soliciting and validating wishes, opinions and choices can help motivate an older person to engage in life and living rather than be pulled into depression and regression.

Time is fleeting ever so swiftly
Don't like me
Don't love me
Just understand me

Leah Cahn

Being a reliable, dependable "other" in the life of a frail older person does not mean that workers can or should attempt to solve all of their problems. Neither does it mean that workers have to like all of their elderly clients.

It is common for workers to feel overwhelmed, helpless and hopeless, just as older people do themselves, by the severity and multiplicity of the losses of their older clients. Older people, struggling with these multiple losses and with basic survival issues can become negative, demanding and oblivious to the feelings of others, including the worker.

Being a reliable and dependable "other" means being there on a regular basis to provide mandated services in a caring and compassionate manner. The time taken for extra listening, the words that show understanding of the older person and his struggle can often be the biggest help of all.

REFERENCES

1. Kaminsky, Marc *What's inside you. It shines out of you.* Horizon Press. New York, 1974.
2. Erikson, Erik *Childhood and Society.* W.W. Norton and Co. 1963 p.260.
3. Kimmel, Douglas *Adulthood and Aging.* John Wiley and Sons, New York. 1980 pp. 332-354.
4. Butler, Robert & Lewis, Myrna *Aging and Mental Health.* C.V. Mosby and Co., Saint Louis 1977 pp.40-43.
   Weisman, Avery *On Dying and Denying* Behavioral Publications, New York. 1972.
5. Butler, Robert & Lewis, Myrna op. cit. pp.61-64.
   Goldfarb, Alvin "Masked depression in the old" Journal of Psychotherapy, Vol. xx1, No.4 Oct. 1967. pp.791-796.
6. Rzetelny, Harriet "Alcohol abuse in Senior Centers" in *Working with the frail elderly in senior centers.* New York State Dept. of Social Services 1981 Available from Brookdale Center on the aging, 440, E. 26th St., NYC.
7. Patterson, Robert "Grief and depression in old people" in Steury and Blank (eds.) *Readings in Psychotherapy with older people.* NIMH, 1979.
8. Butler, Robert and Lewis, Myrna op. cit. p 336, pp.58-61.

Chapter X

Serving the Elderly Blind:
A Generic Approach

Harriet Goodman

INTRODUCTION

When blind people talk with each other about people and institutions outside the network of the visually impaired, they frequently
use the expression "the sighted world." This phrase has a strange
ring for people who take their vision for granted. In their world,
sight is the norm, and they have no need to distinguish themselves
from those who do not see. Yet this expression is common usage
among blind people. It symbolizes the profound separation between
people with severe visual deficits and the community as a whole.
Throughout history, the blind have been set apart as a special group.
Whether they have been scorned and abused or revered for pos-
sessing special insights others lack, in virtually all societies the blind
have been considered different from people with normal sight. They
have always had an unique social role.[1]

Today the specialness of the blind is represented in the elaborate
and costly rehabilitation and social service system designed to assist
the severely visually impaired. It is a network of private and public
agencies and programs which has developed over the past one hundred and fifty years in this country to serve the blind as a separate
group in need. While the proportion of legally blind individuals in
the United States is relatively small, the resources available for the
blind command a good market in the competition for public and
voluntary funds for all disabled people. Other disabilities may affect
a larger segment of the population or may be functionally more
disabling than blindness, yet work for the blind maintains a special
public concern along with a separate service network.[2] These features appear to have endured in spite of efforts to integrate disabled

people into the social and economic mainstream of American life and the increase in public awareness of other disabled groups following the Rehabilitation Act of 1973.

The pool of expertise in work with the blind remains concentrated in specialized agencies. Few helping professionals outside of the blindness system are trained to work with visually impaired people. At the same time, practitioners with the blind continue to stress that their professional colleagues outside the blindness network lack concern and interest, or are perhaps fearful, about working with blind clients.[3] Clearly the complex service structure which has grown up to serve the blind has an interest in its own preservation and enhancement. This desire for organizational maintenance is supported by what Robert A. Scott described as the "sequestering" function of agencies for the blind.[4] The institutional arrangements provided in these services apparently serve a community need to minimize public awareness of blind people. They help to maintain the blind as the unseen in our midst.

This paper addresses the impact of a separate service system for the blind as it affects the largest segment of the visually impaired population, the elderly, and, specifically those people whose visual loss has developed with advancing years. It is directed to practitioners serving older persons in the community who wish to enhance their understanding of this minority group within the aged population. My purpose is to provide workers with a practice perspective which will broaden their knowledge about the impact of vision problems as they intersect the other physical, social and economic losses experienced by older people. In response to the traditional lack of coordination between the aging and blind service networks, I will acquaint the generic worker with deficits in the blindness system as well as the services it offers which can develop social and functional opportunities for the older person. The purpose of this article is to help workers, who encounter older people in the course of their practice, to operate as effective advocates for clients who are experiencing problems with their sight.

THE ELDERLY IN THE BLIND SERVICE SYSTEM

The Scope of the Problem. There is a profound association between visual loss and old age. Changes in visual functioning accompany the aging process. Visual acuity decreases and refractive changes occur, such as increased myopia and astigmatic shift. Advancing years also bring decreased powers of accommodation, diminished ability to adapt to darkness and lowered resistance to glare.[5]

While aging takes a toll on the older person's sensory capacity, the risk of actual blindness and severe visual impairment also increases with age. All of the major diseases of the eye—diabetes, glaucoma, macular degeneration and cataract—are more likely to occur in older people. Even conservative estimates concede that over half of the blind persons in this country are elderly.[6] The American Foundation for the Blind maintains that 65% of all severely visually disabled individuals are over sixty-five, representing over one million individuals.[7] Increased medical knowledge has enabled substantial control of infectious diseases and prenatal influences which can cause blindness in children. At the same time, this country has experienced a demographic shift, increasing the proportion of elderly in our society. Age is the most powerful predictor of the prevalence of blindness and visual impairment.[8] Thus, as older people have higher rates of vision disorders, the number of elderly blind has increased along with the aged population.

The highest incidence of new blindness is among people over sixty-five years with more than half of all new cases of blindness occurring in this age group.[9] As a corollary, most of the blindness in old age is adventitious. It is a new event for people who have lived throughout their lives with normal or correctable vision. Consequently visual deterioration is superimposed on whatever other losses the aging person must integrate and these are likely to be considerable, since most of the elderly blind are poor and are usually over seventy-five years of age.[10]

While it is clear that most of the blind and visually impaired persons in this country are elderly, the actual extent of the aged blind population is unclear. Considerable conflict exists over how blindness should be defined. Advocates for the elderly blind criticize the commonly used definition for legal blindness as biased against impairments found in older people.[11] It is widely assumed that the elderly are more likely to be among the "hidden blind" than other visually disabled persons. They are frequently undercounted and outside the agency service network. Practitioners often cite the reluctance of opthamologists to inform older patients that they are legally blind and they may not register aged people as blind even where legal mandates for such reporting exist. Since the blindness system allocates only 10% of its resources for the benefit of the elderly,[12] the way in which vision problems are defined and the ability of old people to have access to important rehabilitation and social services are interrelated.

Defining Blindness. Although the word "blindness" conjures up the complete absence of vision in the minds of most people, in a social context, the actual definition of blindness represents a range of perceptual losses. A confounding fact to those outside the community of the blind is that only a small percentage, probably one in ten, of those recognized as blind are totally without vision.[13] The variety of capacities of visually impaired people is enormous. Some visually impaired people only have light perception, or the ability to distinguish light and dark while others can discern shapes or colors, travel independently or see normally within a prescribed field of vision. In addressing the Second National Conference on Aging and Blindness in 1976, Dr. August Calenbrander described the visual deficits associated with some of the common eye diseases of old age. They all have very different consequences for the patient's residual sight. The vision loss associated with glaucoma primarily affects side vision. In its advanced stages it leaves an island of relatively unimpaired central vision, commonly called "tunnel vision."[14] With macular degeneration, on the other hand, central vision suffers and peripheral vision remains unaffected. Cataracts result in a general haze over the visual image, similar to a dirty car windshield.[15] These perceptual variations have differential effects on the ability of older people to carry out every day activities.

Individuals also exhibit considerable variation in the degree to which they accommodate their residual vision. With the same objective degree of impairment, some people use their remaining vision in a more productive way than others. Dr. Dan M. Gordon described his clincial experience with 307 elderly patients. He suggested that variables such as age of onset of the impairment, patient attitude and other sensory deficits can affect the functional impact of the disability.[16] To complicate the picture even further, blind clients report fluctuation in their visual acuity. Some days they can see better than others.

The extent of the variation in sensory deficit leads to the problem of deciding who falls into the category of "blind" and who does not and how to properly describe the vast gray area between normal vision and total absence of sight. Along with definition comes the inclusion and exclusion of categories of impaired people, with consequences for who gets served within the blind agency network.

Legal blindness, formulated by the American Medical Association in 1934 is the most widely used classification scheme in the United States.[17] In 1935 it was incorporated into the Blind Title of the Social Security Act and is presently used as the selective basis for eligibility for benefits such as SSI, tax exemption and in some cases sponsorship for rehabilitation training.

This definition sets the parameters for legal blindness where there is (1) central visual acuity of 20/200 or less in the better eye with best correction or (2) a visual field deficit where the widest diameter of the visual field does not subtend to an angle greater than 20°.[18] The Snellen eye chart is used to measure visual acuity. Visual ability of 20/200 is necessary to read the large letter ''E'' on the top of this chart from twenty feet away. The second part of the definition which refers to visual fields means that some blind people can have good central vision, but only in a prescribed range. Although the definition is presumed to be an objective measure, it has been both broadly and narrowly interpreted in different States in which it is used. Also individual opthamologists have been noted to report different findings when examining the same patient.[19]

In addition the definition only accounts for two characteristics of vision—distance acuity and visual fields and ignores other factors which can affect a person's ability to see, such as muscle balance and depth perception. Robert J. Wineburg discusses the impact of this objective measure of blindness on the elderly. While many of the eye problems in old age affect near vision, legal blindness measures distant vision. The legal blindness demarcation grew out of a need to determine standards for employment suitability and is a clinical definition, not based on the functional capacity of a person to utilize his residual vision in the ordinary activities of everyday life. For the retired elderly, it is in the arena of self care and maintenance where the consequences of vision deficits are experienced.[20]

In 1978, Kirchner and Lowman analyzed the sources of variation between two studies of the prevalence of blindness in the United States. These researchers contrasted two data sources from 1970 which produced strikingly different results in the proportion of different age groups identified as blind. The National Center for Health Statistics-Health Interview Survey defined visual disability based on self-report of a person's ability to use his or her sight. This subjective, functional measure of near vision produced an elderly blind population of 68% of all blind persons. In contrast, the Model Reporting Area study using a clinical definition of legal blindness which stressed distance acuity found only 46% of the blind population was over sixty-five. Kirchner and Lowman's findings highlight the impact of the legal blindness definition on the elderly. The definition itself seems to exclude functional manifestations of vision problems experienced by older people. The larger proportion of younger people who are legally registered as blind indicates that the young are more likely to find their way into the service system. It is unclear whether this is because they are more motivated to do so, or because doctors are more consistent in reporting them to the State registries.[21]

The Blind Service Network and the Elderly. In 1969, Robert A. Scott published his now classic sociological study on blindness, *The Making of Blind Men.* A central theme of his work was the inequitable distribution of services for the blind. Scott found that the blind service system focused its resources on children and adult clients with vocational potential. He observed that the elderly, while the majority, did not receive proportionate attention from rehabilitation agencies for the blind. For the most part, services were provided to small numbers of younger clients. The literature in professional journals in the field paralleled this service bias. Few articles existed on the elderly visually impaired.[22]

Also in 1969, the American Foundation for the Blind established a Task Force on Aging and Blindness. In 1972 the Foundation replaced it with an Advisory Committee on Aging. The Committee's purpose was to draw attention to the aged with severe vision problems and develop innovative program approaches for their special needs. The Foundation continues this work, begun a decade ago, to link community services for the elderly and for the blind for their mutual benefit. The Foundation encourages specialized blind agencies to attend to the needs of the elderly blind, and sponsors model projects, such as activities to integrate the visually impaired elderly into the services which proliferated for the elderly following the Older Americans Act.

As Gross points out, Scott's research and the work of the Foundation were attempts to reassess and redirect the traditional service priorities in the field of blindness. The subtle demographic changes taking place in the blind population and the shifting needs of an older blind population with more functional and fewer vocational requirements were recognized. Unfortunately Gross's review of the blindness literature since 1970 indicates little change in service emphasis.[23] Research and practice studies still indicate a preponderance of work with children and working age adults. The limited professional writing on the elderly blind describes program innovations under-taken in recent years, but it provides scant empirical study of older blind people. In fact the service needs of the aged blind still remain undocumented.

Wineburg concludes that the blind service system still emphasizes the productive potential of youth at the expense of the functional and social adaptation of the elderly. He points with equal concern to their exclusion from generic services for the aged and reports the reluctance of community and institutional agencies to serve the elderly blind.[24]

The separation of the aged and blind systems and the residual treatment of elderly with impaired sight is problematic for workers and clients in both service networks. The advantages of cooperative efforts and relevant services for the elderly blind are continually restated at conferences and in papers on aging and blindness. Pro-grams for the aged are concentrations of expertise about resources which can benefit the visually impaired along with the normally sighted older person. Similarly, the blind service agencies are pools of knowledge in solving the special problems of the visually im-paired. The benefits are clear. A skilled practitioner with the blind can train colleagues in the aged service community, mitigating the fear and uncertainty expressed by workers. Increased awareness of vision problems among the elderly can stimulate simple prevention programs, such as glaucoma screening, or increased utilization of treatment and vision service, such as low vision clinics. Many older people experience the loss of vision gradually and accept the impair-ment as "having trouble seeing" and do not seek help. Cooperative efforts between senior services and blind agencies have the potential to promote rehabilitation among large groups of older people who might not recognize the extent of their problems or may not be aware of the restorative potential available through blind agencies.

The search continues for a means of extending services to the elderly with sight problems, whether through the blindness or aging networks or at some intersecting point between the two. Dedication, particularly among blind service professionals, keeps the problem in the forefront. Yet the tradition of separate service and the public's encouragement to keep the blind and the aged hidden work against these efforts. The willingness of the older person identified as blind to withdraw into the protection of the blindness system plagues them as well. Additional factors are the tendency of many older people to minimize vision problems because of the stigma associated with blindness and the social isolation which is the frequent response to sensory loss.

TOWARDS A PRACTICE MODEL FOR THE ELDERLY BLIND

The Impact of Visual Loss in Old Age. Loss and isolation are the intertwined consequences of visual impairment in old age, along with an increase in the older person's need to depend on others. An individual's ability to adapt to his or her loss of eyesight depends on a confluence of environmental circumstances and personal characteristics, as well as the impact of the overall terrain of advancing age. Like the aging process itself, people experience the loss of vision in highly individual ways.

Adventitious blindness is above all a profound sensory loss for a person who has experienced normal vision throughout life. As with any sensory loss, it decreases the pleasure which can be taken in life. Blindness reduces enjoyment from visual appreciation of loved ones, natural beauty and cherished objects. Older people describe it as "living death." Blindness is a blow to one's body image and consequently results in a loss of self-esteem and dignity.

Blindness is a stigmatized condition in our society. Old people carry with them the perceptions which they had earlier in life about the visually handicapped and they frequently integrate them into their new roles as blind people. Like most people, they had considered the blind as helpless, docile and depressed—running a mounting social debt for their dependence on the normally sighted. In some cases they harbored mythological explanations for blindness. As a result they may now consider their loss of vision as punishment for past sins, citing biblical references to document their guilt. Scott pointed out that the visually impaired are socialized to their roles as blind people through interaction with the sighted world.[25] For the adventitiously blind elderly, past perceptions enforce their devaluation, as they assume a new social status.

Frances T. Dover, who for many years coordinated the training of student interns at the New York Jewish Guild for the Blind, reviewed the dynamics of adjustment to visual impairment in adult life. While reactive depression does not always occur, feelings of worthlessness, frustration and anger are often expressed in a pervasive mood which is depressive in character. Typical responses are excessive self-pity, crying, loss of appetite and an inability to sleep. Newly blind people often employ denial and projection as defences against this undesirable situation. Denial can take the form of exaggerated hope that new medical treatment can reverse the condition.[26] Practitioners describe clients who exhaust their financial resources in questionable efforts to regain their sight. "Passing" as sighted is one form of denial which cushions the person from the stigma of disability. While this response is only available to the partially sighted, it helps the person avoid the consequences of an undesirable social status. Many blind older adults continue to deny their disability for many years. This is clearly dysfunctional when it precludes essential help.

The impact of visual deterioration in old age is rarely experienced in isolation. It more often takes place in the context of the cumulative impact of multiple loss which further compromises an older person's ability to utilize remaining strengths and assets. The loss of sight intersects with other physical and mental problems which are common to the aging process. Visual deterioration is associated with a loss of mental functioning, since poor eyesight reduces the ability of external stimuli to elicit appropriate behavior. A study by Snyder et al. of the effects of poor eyesight on mental functioning confirmed that older people with vision problems produced lower scores on a mental status test than older people with normal sight.[27] Unsteady gait and a general loss of physical capacity can frustrate the older blind person's efforts to travel independently.

For the elderly blind, the effectiveness of the other senses may be reduced at the same time there is an increased need to rely on them. In spite of the widespread belief that the blind experience increased acuity in their remaining senses to compensate for their loss of vision, the opposite may hold. For example, neuropathy, or loss of sensitivity in the fingers and toes, may accompany diabetes. The condition can undermine the blind diabetic's efforts to experience the outside world. It can make simple self-care tasks difficult to learn and carry out. Hearing loss, common among older people, is more difficult to accommodate when the person is unable to rely on visual clues. Freedman and Inkster assert that from the older person's point of view, the onset of blindness not only exaggerates other problems of old age, it also increases the person's apprehension about his or her total physical integrity.[28]

The pervasive sense of vulnerability experienced by the aged blind person makes learning new skills for performing daily tasks a problem. Risk taking is difficult and can inhibit efforts to encourage retraining. Vulnerability can also compromise social relationships. It is common for blind people to withdraw from ordinary interactions, as they struggle with their altered relationships with family and friends. Isolation is not only the product of the inaccessibility of social activities, it may protect the person from the oversolicitous response of others and the consequent recognition that one is viewed as dependent and must rely on others for help.

Utilizing Services for the Elderly Blind. Visual impairment has consequences for the older person in two critical life areas—the functional capacity for self care and maintenance and the potential for social interaction and enrichment. These abilities are interrelated and depend to a great deal on each other for their development. A person's ability to adapt to a particular set of physical, economic, social and sensory assaults can affect his or her ability to continue to live in the community. Blindness itself presents a risk in this respect, a fact evidenced by the high proportion of visually impaired persons of all ages in institutional care.[29]

Specialized services for the blind are an important resource to help people continue as closely as possible in their normal life patterns when they lose vision. While blind agencies traditionally emphasize vocational services, they are repositories of skill and expertise in teaching the blind life skills. They may also offer low vision services and opportunities for social interaction. Yet the relative position of the elderly in the blind service system calls for activism and advocacy on the part of workers concerned with the elderly. Workers should learn about particular programs and agencies in their communities which have an interest in older persons with sight problems.[30] The following review is meant to acquaint the generic practitioner with the nature of these services and some of the issues surrounding their utilization by older clients.

Rehabilitation Services. Rehabilitation training provides a blind person with the skills to manage ordinary activities independently and safely. For an adventitiously blind older person, training can help maintain a positive life style in the face of diminished visual acuity. As noted earlier, much of the visual deterioration in old age is a gradual process and older people tend to adapt to vision changes over time. However these coping modes are frequently maladaptive and often unsafe.

Training offers safe and effective methods for carrying out everyday tasks in skills of daily living, mobility and communication. The visually impaired person is taught how to use the remaining senses in order to function without eyesight and in the proper use of specially designed equipment for the blind. Training must be highly individualized in relation to personal needs, abilities and environmental supports and may be directed to very limited goals. Even learning proper sighted guide techniques or the safe method for preparation of hot drinks can significantly affect a person's mastery over the environment. Training has the potential to decrease an older blind person's dependence on family members and neighbors. Apart from the critical issues of personal safety, skills training lessens the need for home care services and long-term care.

It is interesting to note that in New York, the designation, "homemaker," allows the State Commission for the Blind and Visually Handicapped to sponsor activities of daily living instruction for the older blind person who has been registered as legally blind. Mobility and communications training can be offered as adjunct services if necessary. Within the work-based context of the blindness system, "homemaker" in this case is viewed as a vocational goal. The expectation is that helping an older blind person learn proper self-care skills will decrease the need for purchased care. Across the country, many public and private agencies provide rehabilitation service within a generic service context. Some organizations, such as the New York Infirmary's Center for Independent Living, specialize in the rehabilitation needs of people over 55 years of age.

While even limited training for the aged blind is an important service need, it is hampered by the biases of a service network which often considers instruction wasted on the aged. Workers for the blind are not free of societal perceptions about the elderly. They operate for the most part in a system which values the efficiency of their services in relation to productive work or longevity of utilization. Love, for example, points out the lack of knowledge mobility instructors have about the special needs of the older blind client—medical complications, special support aids or even the relevance of mobility instruction. He attributes this gap to the tendency of the blind service system to emphasize work with young, career motivated clients.[31]

Family members and home care providers may also have problems understanding the utility of rehabilitation instruction for the elderly blind. They are likely to view aged blind people as helpless and dependent and it may be difficult for them to conjure up the image of an elderly blind person using a stove, negotiating a city street or signing a check. Such attitudes on the part of people in the trainee's environment complicate the learning process. Those at home may want to take over tasks which the older person can competently perform alone which can intensify the older person's ambivalence about becoming more independent. The problem is further complicated by the fact that the older person, in most cases, does need to depend on others for some tasks. A balance, which can encourage self-reliance while at the same time maintaining the elderly client's ability to ask for and receive needed assistance, is difficult to achieve.

Group Work and Recreational Services. In 1959, Sidney Saul first described segregated groups of elderly blind as an aid in helping older people adjust to visual disability.[32] The impact of a setting where blindness is the norm can be profound for a person facing deteriorating vision. The isolation which plagues the older disabled person is mitigated by social contact with other people who are experiencing similar problems. Group members can become models for a variety of coping styles, which the person can test in relation to his or her own situation. More recently in discussing group services, Emerson and Long employed groups of elderly blind as an arena to voice concerns, clarify values and develop awareness of realistic solutions to problems experienced as disabled people.[33]

Group services often stress the functional adaptation of the older person to his life situation. For example, the New York State Commission for the Blind and Visually Handicapped granted a contract to the Jewish Guild for the Blind to offer group services as a support for older people being trained in skills of daily living. Planning and preparing social events, or working on arts and crafts projects enabled older people in training to rehearse newly learned skills. Clients were stimulated to use nonvisual senses. Within a relaxed social environment, they could test what it was like to engage in a new learning experience late in life.[34]

In spite of proclamations of the value of segregated services within generic agencies for the blind, this method of service delivery is criticized on two counts. Some writers feel generic agencies for the blind discharge their obligations to the elderly by patronizing them. Others feel that such services detract from efforts to integrate programs for the blind and the aged. In many settings, recreational services for older people involve the blind person in passive experiences. They are picked up, fed, entertained and returned home. Rather than use the experience as a model for learning new skills in social and daily living activities, agencies may foster dependence on the part of the older p˅rson.[35] For those who are interested in integration efforts, the blind agency often appears to encourage comfort within a segregated environment, where the blind adult can be protected from the struggle for adequate community service.[36]

Group services are the medium through which efforts to integrate the visually impaired and sighted elderly have developed. The American Foundation for the Blind has widely supported such efforts. Its aim has been to decrease the isolation of the elderly blind at the same time as it increased their utilization of community resources. It has encouraged mainstreaming programs since the 1970's.[37] Efforts focus on bringing older persons to selected community sites. A New York based organization, Vacation and Community Services for the Blind, has undertaken such programs at a remarkable range of local facilities serving the elderly. Although these efforts are frequently met with resistance from organizational and individual participants, they continue to bring about contact between sighted and visually impaired elderly, as well as practitioners from both service systems.

Low Vision Services. The blind agency network is also a resource for services to enhance residual vision for people with poor eyesight. Some individual optometrists and opthamologists have practices in low vision services. Persons with low vision include people with usable vision but whose visual acuity cannot be corrected with normal glasses. Rosenbloom estimates that 20% of the partially sighted population is not seriously impaired enough to qualify as legally blind.[38] This group, as well as legally blind people with residual vision, can frequently benefit from low vision services.

The presence of any remaining vision raises the question as to how that power can be maximized. Low vision aids and equipment which are available as either optical or nonoptical devices offer that potential. Low vision evaluation determines the utility of hand-held or stand magnifiers, telescopes, lamps, visors or large print publications—any device to help people use their vision more efficiently. Rosenbloom and Kelleher stress the importance of seeking specialized low vision services. Most opthamologists lack knowledge about these devices and are not expert in the complicated evaluation and training process required to assure their proper use. A doctor's declaration, "there is nothing more I can do for you," may exclude the restorative potential for functioning that these services offer.[39]

CONCLUSION

This paper has addressed some of the issues in service delivery to older people with vision problems. The visually impaired are a significant minority group within the elderly population, and visual loss is a potential problem for many older clients seen in community services. Neither blind service organizations nor services for the aged adequately concern themselves with this special group. Many older people with sight problems are hidden from these service networks for a variety of reasons. Some elderly people do not appreciate the extent of their eye problems and practitioners with the aged may overlook signs that their clients are experiencing loss of sight. The visually impaired elderly may isolate themselves in response to their eye problems. In some instances services for the normally sighted elderly are inaccessible or may actively exclude blind people. Geriatric workers often assume that blind agencies take care of people with sight problems, but as we have seen the traditional service bias of these organizations leaves the elderly blind inadequately served by this network as well.

Blind agencies continue to avoid their responsibility to make the service community aware of the special problems of the elderly blind and few programs exist to educate community workers in working with sight impaired elderly. Workers are hard pressed to know what to do when they encounter blind people in the course of their practice, let alone how to identify potential vision problems among those who appear to have normal vision.[40] Hopefully this article provides a starting point for the individual worker concerned for the functional maintenance of older people at risk, and will help the practitioner become a better informed advocate for this special group.

REFERENCES

1. Koestler, Frances A. *The Unseen Minority* (New York: David McKay Company, Inc., 1976), pp. 1-3.
2. Lukoff, Irving Faber and Whiteman, Martin *The Social Sources of Adjustment to Blindness* (New York: American Foundation for the Blind, Inc., n.d.), p. 1.
3. Asch, Celine "Training Senior Citizen Centers Staff in Blind Rehabilitation Techniques," *Journal of Visual Impairment and Blindness*, 74 (May 1980): 183-185.
4. Scott, Robert A. *The Making of Blind Men* (New York: Russell Sage Foundation, 1969), p. 93.
5. Rosenbloom, Alfred A. "Care of Elderly People with Low Vision," *Journal of Visual Impairment and Blindness*, 76 (June 1982), pp. 209-210.

6. See for example Corinne Kirchner and Cherry Lowman, "Statistical Briefs: Sources of Variation in Estimated Prevalence of Visual Loss," *Journal of Visual Impairment and Blindness*, 72 (October 1978): 329-333.

7. *Facts About Aging and Blindness* (New York: American Foundation for the Blind, n.d.)

8. Lowman, Cherry and Kirchner, Corinne "Statistical Briefs: Elderly Blind and Visually Impaired Person: Projected Numbers in the Year 2000," *Journal of Visual Impairment and Blindness*, 73 (February 1979): 69-73.

9. *Facts About Aging and Blindness*, op. cit.

10. Wineburg, Robert J. "The Elderly Blind: The Unseen," *Journal of Gerontological Social Work*, 4 (Winter 1981): 55-63.

11. See for example, Kirchner and Lowman, op. cit.; Koestler, op. cit.; and Wineburg, op. cit.

12. Wineburg, op. cit.

13. Calenbrander, August. speech before the Second National Conference on Aging and Blindness, Atlanta, Georgia, March, 1978, Conference Proceedings.

14. A person with normal vision can simulate tunnel vision by looking through a slightly opened fist placed directly in front of one eye.

15. Calenbrander, op. cit.

16. Gordon, Dan M. "Visual Impairment in the Older Patient," *Journal of the American Geriatrics Society*, 15 (November 1967): 1025-1030.

17. *Blindness and Services to the Blind in the United States: A Report to the Subcommittee on Rehabilitation*. National Institute of Neurological Diseases and Blindness, by Donald A. Schon, Project Leader (Cambridge, Massachusetts: OSTI Press, 1968), pp. 17-21.

18. Ibid.

19. Koestler, op. cit., p. 46.

20. Wineburg, op. cit.

21. Kirchner and Lowman, op. cit.

22. Scott, op. cit. and Scott, Robert A. "The Selection of Clients by Social Welfare Agencies: The Case of the Blind," *Social Problems*, 14 (Winter, 1967): 248-257.

23. Gross, Arnold M. "Preventing Institutionalization of Elderly Blind Persons," *Journal of Visual Impairment and Blindness*, 73 (February 1979): 49-53.

24. Wineburg, op. cit.

25. Scott, *The Making of Blind Men*, op. cit., pp. 20-25.

26. Dover, Frances T. "Readjusting to the Onset of Blindness," *Social Casework*, 40 (June, 1959): 334-338.

27. Snyder, Lorraine Haitt; Pyrek, Jane; and Smith, K. Carroll "Vision and Mental Function of the Elderly," *The Gerontologist*, 16 (December, 1976): 491-495.

28. Freedman, S. Saul and Inkster, Douglas E. "The Impact of Blindness in the Aging Process," paper prepared for The Center for Independent Living, New York, December 3, 1976.

29. Kirchner, Corinne and Peterson, Richard "Blind and Visually Impaired Nursing Home Residents: Some Social Characteristics and Services Received," *Journal of Visual Impairment and Blindness*, 74 (December 1980): 401-403.

30. *The American Foundation for the Blind Directory of Agencies Serving the Visually Handicapped in the United States* (New York: American Foundation for the Blind, 1981) is an invaluable guide in locating regional resources for the blind. It is available in the reference section of many libraries or may be purchased directly from the AFB by writing to their Publications Department; 15 West 16th Street; New York, New York 10011.

31. Love, James "Orientation and Mobility Problems among the Geriatric Blind Population: A Survey of Need," *Journal of Visual Impairment and Blindness*, 76 (February 1982): 66-68.

32. Saul, Sidney R. "Group Work with Blind People," *New Outlook for the Blind*, 53 (February 1959): 58-60.

33. Emerson, Donna L. and Long, Marla "Interagency Cooperation in an Adult Discussion Group for Visually Impaired Older People," *Journal of Visual Impairment and Blindness*, 72 (January 1978):15-19.

34. Goodman, Harriet "The Elderly Blind: Group Work as a Support for Rehabilitation Training," paper presented at the Second Annual Group Work Conference, Arlington, Texas, April, 1980.

35. Freedman and Inkster, op. cit.

36. Freid, Jacob "The Blind Senior Citizen's Needs," *The Braille Monitor*, (March/April 1977): 110-112.

37. *How to Integrate Aging Persons Who Are Visually Handicapped into Community Senior Programs* (New York: American Foundation for the Blind, n.d.)

38. Rosenbloom, op. cit.

39. Kelleher, Dennis K. "Orientation to Low Vision Aids," *Journal of Visual Impairment and Blindness*, 73 (May 1979): 161-166 and Rosenbloom, op. cit.

40. Another useful publication from the AFB is *An Introduction to Working with the Aging Person Who is Visually Handicapped.* It offers concrete and useful information about managing personal contacts with blind people. It gives some information about special services for the elderly. It is also available from the Publications Department of the AFB.

Chapter XI

Social Work With Elderly Alcoholics: Some Practical Considerations

David Sumberg

As a nation we seem to deal with our elderly population in ways more suited to the production of commodities than to the well-being of humans. Applying, as we often do, the rules and values of the marketplace to our old people, we tend to discard them just as we do any goods from which we no longer derive any profit. The attitudes implicit in such behavior are also implicit in the negative stereotyping of the aging as feeble, dependent, and inadequate. In the case of the elderly who are alcoholic, the error is compounded. Moral judgments that are part of our Puritan culture and are reinforced by our national history only serve to exacerbate already distorted and prejudiced views. It is clear that social work faces a serious and important challenge in its approach to the treatment of alcoholics who are also senior citizens.

This paper attempts to outline the parameters of the problem as well as suggest some practical treatment approaches.

Alcoholics have traditionally been considered the "refuse" of our society—a view best summed up in the public's image of the "skid row" figure. Since the days of early industrialization we have taken a moral approach to alcoholism treatment—exemplified by the axe-wielding Carrie Nation and her cohorts. Other attempts to cope with the problem invoked the basic laws of the land—as in the Prohibition Era—in our dealings with alcoholics. In many states to this day the law and the Women's Christian Temperance Union still hold their original sway. It is only recently, as the economic costs of alcoholism to business and government, including in particular the military, have risen to alarming proportions that society has set out to study the problem on any scale. Even so, current concern is focused mainly on the working or potentially working alcoholic.

The aging have, for the most part, been excluded from the research that receives funding.

It is not surprising, therefore, to discover that the extent of alcohol abuse among older people has not been properly measured. For one, definitions of terms—"elderly" as well as "alcohol abuse"—not only vary but manage to create confusion. Some researchers have chosen 50 years as the onset of old age, assuming that the following three decades or so reveal the indicia. Others use well-marked changes in life, for example, retirement, to distinguish the period.[1]

Similarly there is a wide range of definitions for alcohol abuse. Measurements of the quantity of alcohol consumed are juxtaposed against factors of gender, socioeconomic conditions, and life situations.[2] Many studies show a decrease in amount consumed for all age groups over 50.[3] What needs to be pointed out, however, is that the amount of alcohol consumed has little to do with the issue of problem drinking. A single drink may often precipitate behavior that is thoroughly destructive to the individual, the family, friends, and the social matrix. Again, those indicators of alcoholism in a younger person, such as, for example, losing jobs, family, friends, would not necessarily apply to the elderly for whom these events can be considered normal consequences of aging.

Despite the ambiguity of definitions that still plagues much of the research, it is possible to discern the magnitude of the problem. In community-based studies the incidence of alcoholism among the elderly has been reported as between 2 and 10 percent.[4] Studies of older patients in general or psychiatric hospital wards show a range of alcohol-related problems of 15 to 49 percent.[5] From these two types of studies alone, it is clear that alcoholism and/or problem drinking affects a sizable number of elderly people. If we take the over-65-year-old group, estimated at 12 percent of the population now and at 17 percent by the second decade of the next century,[6] and we further assume a 10 percent rate of alcoholism, we are talking conservatively of about 2½ million elderly people suffering from the disease of alcoholism. We also now know from clinical experience that this group is a heterogeneous one: rich and poor, white and nonwhite, men and women.[7]

Three main styles of alcoholic drinking have been encountered in the field. The chronic alcohol abuser has been drinking alcoholically through middle age and continues the alcoholic drinking into old age. The reactive drinker in responding to loss e.g., jobs, wife-husband roles, or loved ones—loses control of the drinking, passes an "imaginary line," and develops the disease of alcoholism. Finally, there is the binge drinker who is able to maintain abstinence or social drinking behavior for long periods of time between short bursts when the drinking goes out of control. Each of these three types, of course, presents special treatment issues to social workers. Each is also well represented among the elderly alcoholic population.

ISSUES IN TREATMENT

The social worker who attempts to deal with elderly alcoholics must become especially sensitized to those aspects of the disease and its therapy that are peculiar to this group. He/she must first deal with the challenge implied in the basic question—Why try to help them stop drinking at all? For so many of the elderly, drinking would appear to be one of life's few remaining pleasures. As so many old people are afflicted with the fear of approaching death,[8] it would be cruel to deprive them of the release offered by alcohol. Such an argument confuses the effects of social drinking with those of alcoholism. Most often social drinking in the elderly results in increased social interaction, an anesthetizing effect on bodily pains and aches, and mild feelings of well-being. For the alcoholic, however, the results are never benign. An alcoholic by definition has no control over alcohol: a single drink produces subtle and profound changes in his physical, mental, emotional and social life.

To the elderly alcoholic, that one drink can be particularly devastating. What starts out as increased social interaction turns often into isolation and guilt. The anesthetizing effect eventually masks brain, liver, and kidney damage resulting from the toxic nature of alcohol. The sense of well-being is converted into self-doubt and self-hatred.

Another issue facing the social work professional is the notion that alcoholics are hopeless cases. An alcoholic can never cure his disease; he can only arrest it by stopping the drinking. The disease lies dormant while he/she abstains from drinking, to be awakened to the original—or even higher—level of severity by the first drink. A particularly frustrating aspect of this chronicity is the regression in total functioning after the resumption of drinking. When the social worker sees months of work destroyed by a single drink, it is understandable that he or she may consider the alcoholic as hopeless.

With the elderly alcoholic it is especially easy to blame the "entrenched lifetime personality structure" for the drinking rather than the disease itself.

Perhaps the most frustrating aspect of working with the elderly alcoholic is denial. Denial, shared by all alcoholics, young or old, is a factor basic to all addiction. The compulsion created by the disease is stronger than all the reasons for not drinking. And with the elderly their very status may provide additional rationale for indulgence. They may need to deny approaching death. The social worker, recognizing this need, will sometimes strengthen this denial in order to enhance the client's strength in fighting physical illness and spiritual despair. The social worker may also unconsciously be trying to deal with his/her own feelings about death and loss. But normal denial-of-death mechanisms become destructive when coupled with the denial that is tied into the disease of alcoholism. The elderly alcoholic, who repeatedly finds "reasons" for drinking, short-circuits the worker's need to address the issues around dying. For the alcoholic, thematic work centering on dying becomes all the more "reason" to drink. The effect on social workers in seeing their "work" used as a reason to drink is often anger at the client and confirmation that the elderly alcoholic is hopeless.

Another source of conflict in working with the aged alcoholic concerns loss. Many social workers feel ambivalent about asking an aged client who is normally facing loss of friends, family, job, role, and status to face another loss—the bottle. Many alcoholics will tell social workers, "The bottle is the only comfort left. Don't make me lose that too!" In fact what is really occurring in alcohol abuse is a blockage in the formal grieving process. The social worker who helps the aged alcoholic grieve the loss of the bottle paradoxically helps the alcoholic learn to cope with other losses in life. The worker in effect is helping the alcoholic not so much to lose the bottle but to gain life again.

WHAT IS TO BE DONE

Each social worker and social work agency should make the commitment to do outreach and education not only with the elderly themselves but with those individuals, community organizations, and tenant groups, in both public and private housing that are likely to be concerned with the problems of the elderly alcohol abuser.

The police, doctors, hospital employees, family and friends, who may have frequent contact with the elderly alcohol abuser need information and instruction in how to recognize signs of problem drinking, training in how to motivate the client to accept help, and knowledge of available resources. Such education, whether for the elderly or others, must be undertaken with tact. Negative attitudes toward alcoholics need to be both elicited and gently confronted. The most successful education about alcoholism and its effects on the older person is probably carried out by a recovered elderly person in conjunction with a social worker trained in alcoholism education. The evidence of hope embodied in the recovered person and the social worker's knowledge of what to do and where to go for help proves an effective combination. Perhaps, most effective of all is the use of self-help groups made up of peers who understand what the alcoholic is experiencing.

Community organizers can play an important role, particularly in work with retirement communities where heavy drinking has become the norm. Here the community becomes the client: education, diagnosis, and self-help can provide a significant contribution to alcoholism work.

TREATMENT

Identifying the Alcoholic

The first step in helping elderly alcohol abusers is to identify and bring into treatment those in need of help. Once the at-risk person is identified, the social worker should ascertain current drinking patterns, explore any history of drinking and watch for signs which might indicate alcohol abuse. Social workers must learn to make detailed explorations of drinking behavior a regular part of their interview techniques. Direct questions work best.

—How much do you drink each day?
—Have you ever had a period of time while drinking when you functioned but had no memory of it (blackouts)?
—Has a doctor ever told you not to drink? What did you do?
—Have you ever lost a job? Why?
—Have you ever decided to stop drinking? Why?
—Have you ever wanted to stop but couldn't?

These questions as well as many others can be found in Alcoholics Anonymous (AA) literature obtainable from local AA groups and the local chapters of The National Council on Alcoholism. Other local groups dealing with alcoholism may also be a source of information on diagnosis as well as treatment.

Other signs of alcoholism in the elderly are insomnia, accidents leading to fractures, bruises, etc., suicide attempts, history of sexual malfunctioning, sudden onsets of organic brain syndrome, and sudden, destructive changes in behavior that have no other discernible cause. These symptoms, of course, can be caused by other old age problems but if they are present they should at least be explored for possible alcohol-related connections.

A good nose is also a help in identifying elderly alcohol abusers. On the evidence of smell alone, it is important to ask clients about their pattern of drinking. Social workers are often embarrassed to do so and the alcoholic may play on this embarrassment in order to hide his or her drinking. So it is essential to be forthright on the evidence of the social worker's sense of smell.

Social workers should also be alert to the responses they get from an elderly alcohol abuser. As has already been noted, one aspect of the disease of alcoholism is denial of the effects of drinking in the face of obvious evidence to the contrary. Unfortunately, this type of denial often leads to feelings of frustration and anger on the part of the worker. Any expression of such feelings often provides the alcoholic with a perverse pleasure and an additional rationale to reinforce the addiction. He or she is saying in effect, "Another person who doesn't understand me! The only thing that helps me is my bottle!" The social worker needs to recognize denial as an unconscious process which is a result of the disease itself.

The importance of careful assessment of responses to questions about drinking behavior can be best illuminated by an apocryphal story from the field. It seems that a social worker asked a client, who had originally sought help for depression because her family had "rejected" her, "how much she had been drinking?" The client replied that at most she had two drinks a night. Since this was less than the social worker himself drank many evenings, he assumed the woman had no alcohol-related problems. But being naturally suspicious he asked again how many drinks she consumed a day. Over and over, she replied "two." Finally the social worker asked her what size the glasses were. It turned out that the "two" drinks were eight ounce water tumblers filled to the top with vodka!

Equally significant was the worker's next question: "What happens to you when you drink?" What followed was a description of severe behavioral change following the two drinks. She became morose and would lash out in anger at the family members who were trying to help her, rejecting all their efforts to care for her yet berating them for their "non-caring" feelings. The connection between the presenting problem and the drinking might have been lost if the social worker had not actively pursued the details in the client's more generalized answers.

Encouraging Recognition by the Client

Once problem drinking has been identified, workers must help their clients understand the connection between the onset of their psychological pain, and physical ailments and the consumption of alcohol. For alcoholics these pains are often the *result* of drinking, not the *cause* of the drinking. In fact, searching for a "prime cause" in alcohol abuse is largely a dead-end route in alleviating alcoholism. In his clinical work this author has found it futile even for those elderly problem drinkers who could be classified as "reactive drinkers." It would seem logical that if the primary stress was dealt with at the beginning of treatment, a person could return to social drinking. What usually happens, however, is that as we search for reasons for the drinking or start the process of examining the "cause" of the client's problems, drinking itself undermines the therapeutic benefit of our work.

Alcoholics Anonymous suggests that the first step towards recovery is the admission by the drinker that he or she has become powerless over alcohol and that the drinker's life has become unmanageable. For the elderly alcoholic, as for most alcoholics, this admission is a particularly difficult one to make in the face of the strong denial component of the disease. Paradoxically, alcoholics are also convinced that through the use of alcohol, they *gain control* over their lives. The alcohol, they believe, makes them less lonely, less depressed, wittier and altogether more successful. Thus, social workers would seem to be asking elderly alcoholics to do without the one thing that gives them some control over the pain and anxieties of their lives. How then do social workers deliver the message that drinking is the cause of their troubles rather than the cure?

Certainly, the first task is to educate the client as to the physical, emotional, and spiritual effects of alcohol. All social workers in gerontology need to learn at least the rudiments of alcoholism education. Many elderly people who are abusing alcohol feel intense shame and guilt over their drinking. Part of this is an aspect of the disease itself, but part is associated with belonging to a generation raised to consider drinking as either a problem of will power (no will is involved once the disease is activated) or a sin (the implicit free will issue). This is best understood if we think of a sober alcoholic having the free will to pick up the first drink but not the second, third, or the hundredth. Conversely, free will in sobriety is connected to the acceptance of one's powerlessness over alcohol.

Dealing with Denial

Another task is to deal with the client's denial system. Social workers, frustrated over repeated denials of the effects of the drinking, may feel impelled to use the drinking behavior or resulting problems as clubs to beat the client into sobriety. An example of this mechanism is exemplified by two cases known to the author. In one the client's liver was so deteriorated from drinking that he was advised to have a renal shunt. After the operation it was exasperating to hear the client declare that the need for the operation was caused by the "impurities" in the vodka, not the drinking per se! Another client, age 67, after ten years on the Bowery and repeated detoxifications, insisted that he was being hospitalized for the eighteenth time because he wasn't eating when he drank. In both cases the social worker tried to scare his clients with their medical problems. It is a rule of thumb in the field that "you can't scare an alcoholic."

The social worker must listen to the denial, point out the error in the thinking, and guard against getting involved in argument. He or she must make it clear that while he or she can understand the client's need to justify the drinking, still it is the drinking that is causing pain and anguish and there is a way to make life better. Even if clients persist in arguing, they will have heard the message that hope is realistic and help is available.

It is vital for social workers to accept and keep in mind the simple fact that many alcoholics will continue drinking in spite of the worker's efforts. To avoid the natural reaction of frustration, social workers should focus on those in their caseload who actually begin taking steps towards recovery. The elderly alcoholic who tries to cut down this week needs help in order to keep trying after the week is over. We realize readily that our time and strength are limited, but we should recognize that we are also "powerless over the alcohol" in our clients' lives. We can, however, have greater chance of success when we help those who take that first step and put the cork back in the bottle.

Many times elderly alcoholics approach social work agencies, day centers, health facilities, etc. for services not directly connected with their alcoholism. They may be suffering from health problems, loss of housing, and loss of jobs. They may simply be feeling the need to leave behind something that matters, a mark on the world that they have existed. For some, a reconciliation or disengagement with their families has become urgent. These issues are important for the elderly client and as such should of course be addressed. However, the denial system used by alcoholics may focus on these issues to prevent recognition of the drinking. Workers, if they suspect problem drinking, should gently refocus the interview on the interplay between the issue stated by the client and the drinking behavior. In this way, clients are made to realize from the outset that the worker recognizes their social functioning has probably been negatively affected by their drinking.

Meeting Concrete Needs

Other early interventions should include helping the elderly alcoholic with his or her concrete needs. For example, arranging transportation is often essential if treatment is to be conducted in a clinic setting. The availability of food, coffee, or cigarettes gives the message that the social worker and the agency care. Most alcoholics are essentially deprived people and having their needs immediately gratified helps toward establishing a working alliance speedily. The author often keeps a bowl of candy on his desk for this purpose. Along with transportation and food, medical care should be attended to promptly. Many alcoholic clients suffer from severe vitamin deficiencies caused by the drinking. Often symptoms looking like Korsakoff's Syndrome are vitamin deficiencies which can be corrected. It is particularly urgent to have doctors available who are educated about the disease of alcoholism as it effects elderly people. Most elderly people need medications, many of which often have a synergistic effect with alcohol requiring the attention and experience of a doctor trained in alcoholism work. Furthermore, decisions about the use of psychotropic medicines and Disulfarum (antabuse) may have to be made. Other concrete issues which might be addressed concern housing, clothing, and finances, though, it must be emphasized, never at the expense of sobriety work.

Monitoring Recovery

Social workers must be prepared to monitor constantly whether the client is using the treatment for meeting his or her concrete needs exclusively. If the client continues to drink, then in effect, we aid and enable the alcoholism by helping him or her to live more comfortably.

We must continually ask the elderly alcoholic if he or she is willing to stop drinking at once. In fact, it is often useful to ask at the outset if he or she can stay sober for one day, 24 hours from the time of the interview. Most alcoholics with even a modicum of motivation will try it even if only to "prove" to the social worker that they can "control" their drinking. The day-at-a-time concept which should be reinforced by the social worker at the end of each day is particularly applicable to treatment of the elderly person who, in fact, may be living a day at a time.

Support Services

Many recovering elderly alcoholics would benefit from vocational and recreational therapy. A person who is drinking chronically or drinking reactively is suffering from lowered self-esteem caused by toxic effect of the alcohol on the nervous system. Even people who have a positive self-view often suffer in their attitudes toward their selves after too many drinks the night before. In the case of older people, the social loss of esteem due to forced retirement because of age or because of the drinking is added to the psychological loss. One factor which can reinforce sobriety is the positive feeling developed from actively pursuing individual interests. Workers should patiently ask recovering elderly alcoholics what interests, dreams, hobbies, and work goals they have perhaps entertained but have not yet reached. Two examples from the author's caseload will illuminate this point.

Ralph, a 70-year-old recovering alcoholic, during a session, when the issue of interests was raised, revived a childhood interest in the saxophone. This delightful black man, with the help of the worker, entered a music school and began learning how to play. For him, playing the saxophone gave a new focus to hours that had previously been spent alone with his bottle.

Another client, a 62-year-old white male from the New York City Bowery, decided that he still wanted to work. He found a job as a janitor, found himself a girlfriend and lived the last five years of his life quite sober, happy, and busy.

It is important for social workers not to yield to the stereotyped thinking that the elderly alcoholic is "finished" with life. For many alcoholics, sobriety becomes the start of their lives. It is the social worker's task then to help define and support their client's new life goals.

The social worker should also be steering the client in the direction of support groups. These groups may be self-help groups like Alcoholics Anonymous, social group work sessions, family therapy and/or community groups. One of the hallmarks of alcohol abuse is isolation. Alcohol cuts off the drinker from realistic interactions with others. Alcohol also releases social inhibitions that weigh relationships with too much need or too much anger. If we add the effects of the isolation caused by the disease to the normal losses experienced in old age, groups become a viable means of recovery for this population. The group distributes attachment feelings among a larger base of people which cushions future loss. Gains in self-respect engendered by the group's acceptance of the elderly alcoholic will more than offset any of the negative results from encouraging an older person to attach to others who may die soon. Mixed-age groups might also be helpful as long as the specific needs of the elderly members become the group's concern as well. Perhaps the main reason groups are especially useful in treating the elderly alcoholic is that they can reestablish a health-oriented social matrix, one that reinforces sober living and supports newly-awakened growth.

Dealing With Loss of Alcohol

A vital issue in treatment is loss.[9] It has been well documented how significant the dynamics of loss are in the life of the elderly population. Elderly clients are often grieving, denying losses, or expecting more losses. Social workers working with an elderly population must address these issues. For the elderly alcoholic still another loss needs to be addressed by the social worker—the loss of alcohol. Whether it has been used many years or used only since a grievous shock, alcohol often becomes the "best friend" of the drinker. It "helps me forget," "makes me feel good," "helps me feel like a human being." When the recovering elderly alcoholic puts down the drink, he or she will experience it as another loss. This loss should be discussed openly with the client in the social worker's effort to help the client to grieve. One should not, however, dwell on the loss especially during the initial stage of treatment. An acknowledgement of the loss coupled with a renewed focus on the positive aspects of the sobriety is often most helpful in recovery work.

Above all, treating the elderly alcoholic client requires faith on the part of the worker that recovery from alcoholism is possible. Such faith can feed the recovery of an alcoholic as nothing else can. How do social workers find this faith? We need to educate ourselves about the disease of alcoholism and its impact on elderly clients. We need to support one another in staff meetings, supervision, and discussion, recognizing that the immense scope of the problem does not lend itself to easy answers. Most of all, we need to learn from those elderly alcoholics who have recovered and can share a vision of what can be. When workers are properly fed, their elderly clients will be able to draw from them the sustenance they need in their struggle for recovery from the disease of alcoholism.

REFERENCES

1. Duckworth, Grace and Rosenblatt, Adylin "Helping the Elderly Alcoholic," *Social Casework* (May, 1976), p.296.
Rathbone-McCuan, Eloise and Triegaardt, Jean "The Older Alcoholic and the Family," *Alcohol Health and Research World*, 3, No. 4 (Summer, 1979), p.7.
Rosin, Arnold and Glatt, M.M. "Alcohol Excess in the Elderly," *Quarterly Journal of Studies on Alcohol*, 32(1971), p.53.
Cited in Gomberg, E. "Drinking and Problem Drinking Among the Elderly," *Alcohol, Drugs and Aging: Usage and Problems* (Institute of Gerontology, University of Michigan), p.2.
2. Ibid., pp.3-14.
3. Cited in Mayer, M. "Alcohol and the Elderly: A Review," *Health and Social Work*, 4, No.4(November 1979), p.132.
4. Bailey, M., Haberman, P. and Aikshe, H. "The Epidemiology of Alcohol in an Urban Residential Area," *Quarterly Journal of Studies on Alcohol*, 26(March, 1965), pp.19-40.
5. Gomberg, E. op.cit., pp.8-9.
6. Mayer, M. op.cit.,p.131.
7. Gomberg, E. op.cit.,pp.3-14.
8. Monk, A. "Social Work with the Aged: Principles of Practice," *Social Work* (January, 1981), p.61.
9. Goldberg, M. "Loss: A Major Dynamic in the Treatment of Alcoholism," Paper presented at the N.A.S.W. 12th Annual All Alcoholism Conference. Fordham University, New York City 1980, pp.1-2.

Chapter XII

The Holocaust Survivor in Late Life

The term Holocaust refers to the extermination of six million Jews during the Nazi era 1933-45. It was a gradual process of genocide systematically and meticulously implemented while the world stood by and did nothing to stop it. Every Jew in Nazi occupied Europe—which included all European countries except England and Sweden was doomed to death. This was the official Nazi policy.

For four decades since the end of World War II, the Holocaust was a taboo subject. Society at large showed no interest in this unbelievable human event in recent history and survivors responded by silence. Whether they could not or would not talk there was no one to listen.

Within the last few years we have witnessed a sudden and continuing interest in the subject. Public awakening of consciousness about the Holocaust also led to an interest in its survivors—a unique group of people among the aging and aged in our society.

We do not know much about this population but whatever knowledge is available should be shared. Firstly the shared knowledge may enhance our sensitivity and competence in the delivery of service to Holocaust survivors whose advanced age brings them into the orbit of geriatric facilities in our communities, particularly in the larger metropolitan areas.

Holocaust related knowledge also furthers our understanding of survivor children—the Second Generation—who increasingly tend

This paper was presented at the annual conference of the North East Gerontology Society held in Newport, R.I., in May, 1983 and is partly based on the author's article in *Social Casework*, April, 1983, "Implications of the Holocaust for Social Work."

© 1985 by The Haworth Press, Inc. All rights reserved.

to identify themselves as "heirs" to the Holocaust and want to be understood within this perspective.

Furthermore, while the Holocaust is unique, it does bear similarities to other and current genocidal events around the globe. Victims of these man-made calamities are increasingly visible in our communities and deserve a recognition of the massive trauma they have experienced as a result of the destructive events. The literature on Holocaust survivors—despite its imperfections—offers valuable insights into the long-term effects of such traumatization and the impact on generations that follow.

Even more important is to harness the unique contribution survivors can make in transmitting their personal knowledge about genocide and survival. These lessons must be studied, assimilated and applied to prevent the recurrence of another such massive disaster. The world can ignore the lessons of the Holocaust "only at its peril."[1]

At a recent commemorative mass gathering of Holocaust survivors in the nation's capital many speakers highlighted the vital contribution made by survivors in keeping the memory of the Holocaust alive and continuing to remind the world that "the line between barbarism and civilization is thin and needs constant watching."[2]

LESSONS OF THE HOLOCAUST

What does the Holocaust teach and what can we learn from its survivors?

The major lesson of the Holocaust is that it has happened and that it can happen again. "It enters the realm of the possible and is eminently repeatable given the current confluence of circumstances."[3] A systematic study of the Nazi genocide against the Jews provides crucial lessons for today and all times.

The lessons taught by the Holocaust are about the consequences of blind conformity to authority and abdication of individual responsibility; about the danger inherent in the breakdown of democracy; about the tragic consequences of racial politics, about the potential for destruction as a consequence of technological buildup and the perversion of modern languages to conceal murderous objectives.

The Holocaust confronts us with the truth that professional competence and skill are hollow and even dangerous, unless embodied in human values. In Nazi Germany, outstanding judges participated in writing the racial laws, experienced physicians conducted gruesome human experiments, and the best engineers built the chambers for extermination.[4] Professionals whose lives are devoted to healing of psychic wounds and understanding complexities of human behavior can find significant lessons in the study of the Holocaust.

It teaches about the limitless human capacity for cruelty and endurance; about the infinite range of behaviors and coping humans are capable of even in environments of hell, and about the effects of massive traumatization, not only on the victims, but on generations that follow. The study of survivors whose childhood was spent in death camps invites challenges to our theories of human development and provokes the search for new vistas of knowledge.

HOLOCAUST-SURVIVORS—WHO ARE THEY?

Holocaust survivors are Jews who came to this country in two emigration waves: in the 1930's as victims of the Nazi persecution and in the late 1940's as survivors of the "Final Solution." With the outbreak of World War II and the Nazi take over of the European continent, each Jew was doomed to death. Survivors of the "Final Solution" are individuals who outlived the Nazi extermination program and were miraculously found alive by the allied liberation forces in 1945. It is estimated that of the over six million Jews who had lived in Europe before World War II about 500,000 survived.

We know little about Holocaust survivors—despite the fact that they have lived among us for four decades. While a body of psychological literature has developed, much of it is repetitive. Even bare demographic facts are unavailable.

Since the Nazi extermination policy called for immediate destruction of the children and the old, only a very small number of either group was among the surviving remnant. Hence, the majority were in their twenties or thirties at the time of their liberation, and those still alive are currently aging or aged. This is one of the few "hard" facts we do have about this population.

There is another well established fact: survivors are not a homogeneous group. While all have in common the Holocaust experience, they differ markedly in economic, religious, ideological and psychological characteristics. This diversity may be rooted in the heterogeneity of the *now totally extinct* Jewish communities of Europe in which survivors and their ancestors had lived before the Holocaust. Survivors' values, behaviors, aspirations and expectations of their children and of societal institutions may be deeply embedded in these pre-Holocaust experiences.

Therefore, anyone working with this population must have some familiarity with Jewish life in Europe before the destruction.[5] Similarly, the opportunities and limitations encountered by survivors in the years and decades after liberation must be taken into consideration as we aim to understand and respond to the needs of this aging group of people.

THE HOLOCAUST EXPERIENCE

The Holocaust experience itself is also more diversified than most people realize. While many survivors had the experience of internment in Nazi Concentration Camps and Death Camps, there were other "hellish" environments from which survivors crawled out at the time of liberation. These included hiding places, sometimes not larger than a closet in an apartment or a haystack in a barn; or the experience of living in forests as partisan fighters. Some managed to stay alive by concealing their identity and trying to pass as "Aryans."

Each of these environments contained unique stresses and brought forth unique coping mechanisms which may still reverberate in the lives of survivors and their offspring. All lived for years in constant terror of detection, blackmail and arrest. If caught they were subjected to the cruelest forms of punishment before being put to death as a "lesson" to the yet undetected others who were daring to fool the Nazi authorities.[6]

Life and death in the Ghettos and Camps are well documented. The reality of these infernos included starvation diets, along with requirements for heavy labor, total degradation to the point of dehumanization, recurrent terror of selection for the crematoria, and never knowing whether one would be allowed to live another day.

Imprisonment in the Concentration Camp was often preceded by loss of family members in the ghettos, or involved the excruciating experience of separation on arrival in the camp, since parents, wife and children were immediately sent to the gas chambers for extermination.[7]

How did people cope with such enormous and protracted trauma? There is well established evidence that prisoners differed in their response to these extraordinary experiences. Many developed "psychic numbing," a form of extreme emotional detachment which helped them get through the day of hard labor, hunger and terror.

The coping behaviors of others might include extreme selfishness, even cruelty toward fellow inmates, a defense described as "identification with the aggressor." There were prisoners who walked around like "Zombies," totally indifferent to their surroundings and the imminent threat of death.[8]

Astonishingly, we find that even in this substratum of existence there were instances of self-sacrifice, fundamental human decency and altruism.

There were prisoners who shared their starvation diets, cared for the sick and consoled the bereaved. Under the most brutal conditions many kept diaries, wrote poems and created art, depicting the reality of a world of agony in the hope that these materials would survive and tell the world what happened.[9] There is also evidence that morale and adaptive behavior were greatly enhanced by the existence of a supportive relationship. . . "The pair was the basic unit of survival."[10] And yet, it is important to remember that none of these psychological or social supports really mattered in insuring eventual survival. The Gestapo and only the Gestapo determined who would live and who would die, and more accurately, *when* one would die. Under the weight of thousands of chronicles and documentaries, the vital role of accident in biological survival is clearly established as a historic fact. The notion that one survived merely because of ego strength is false. The experience of those who remained alive after the mass murders in Vietnam and Cambodia also supports this basic fact.

Long-Term Effects

What are the long-term effects of living for years in environments, appropriately described as the "Kingdom of Death"?[11]

By and large survivors have evidenced a wide range of adjustments in the years and decades that followed the Holocaust. Some have never recovered from the massive assaults on their body and soul and continued to be plagued by physical and emotional after affects. Gastrointestinal and arthritic conditions, migraine headaches associated with Holocaust related experiences of starvation, cramping in the hiding places and head injuries as a result of beatings have been observed in many Holocaust survivors.

Some have suffered chronic states of anxiety, depressive moods, excessive guilt and even nightmares and flashbacks of genocidal content. Curiously, these problems did not appear immediately but after years, even decades, following the traumatization.[12]

Appropriately or inappropriately clinical observations of post-Holocaust psychopathology have been later applied to victims of wars, revolutions or hostage situations—considered to be "outside the range of usual human experiences." The DSM III new classification of "Post-traumatic Stress Disorders" reflects this clearly and the problems of the Vietnamese veteran are often perceived within this context.[13]

It should be noted that many survivors of the Holocaust were not affected by these post-traumatic disorders. Many, perhaps the majority, have managed to integrate into society as functioning individuals. Many have shown extraordinary energy in creating new lives, achieving economic independence, raising wholesome families and making contributions to society at large.

How this was possible we do not know since stress of such colossal nature would be expected to leave permanent and severe scars on all.

Unfortunately no research has focused on identifying those adaptive integrative forces that facilitated survivors in their process of rebirth and reintegration.

Did preexisting personality and value system play a role? Did successful coping with extreme stress enhance adaptive capacities? Did meaning attached to survival make a difference?

This final question deserves particular attention in our deliberations on issues relevant to aging. One of the themes echoed by many survivors and writers in this field suggests that the degree of the post-Holocaust adjustment was contingent upon reestablishing a sense of purpose in life which incorporated a meaningful expression of their survivorship.[14]

This might take on a variety of forms, such as creating new families to replenish the losses; engaging in humanitarian or religious activities; supporting the State of Israel; involvement in antinuclear programs or organizing and participating in activities that keep the knowledge of the Holocaust alive.

IMPLICATIONS FOR PRACTICE AND RESEARCH

The need for a purpose in life as an effort to master the extreme sorrow and inner chaos resulting from confrontation with the senseless, destructive experiences of the Holocaust is considered to be a key survivor task, the resolution of which may affect how survivors will cope with the process of aging.[15] This is a hypothesis worth exploring and testing, given the uniqueness of an aging population in which each individual has outlived a sentence of death and an immersion in "the end of the world experience."[16] The study of Holocaust Survivors may offer other insights into the world of aging. One of the striking facts about this population is a lack of role models for aging in their family backgrounds. Holocaust survivors have not seen their parents grow to an old age. The mothers and fathers were often killed in the fourth or fifth decade of their lives. While all Jews were meant to die and indeed most were eventually annihilated, the parental generation of the current survivor was selected for death immediately and precisely because its middle-age marked the generation as old and useless even for free labor as slaves.

As advanced age and declining illness now bring survivors into contact with hospitals, nursing homes and institutions for the aged, there is need for an understanding and relatedness to the particular issues, practical and dynamic, that stem from the extraordinary trauma each of these individuals has experienced in his/her earlier life.

Some of these issues are highlighted below.

Vulnerability to Loss and Illness

Holocaust survivors may have a particular vulnerability to experiences inherent in the process of aging, such as loss, separation, illness or institutionalization. Because there was no opportunity to grieve or mourn during these catastrophic years, an experience of extreme stress may elicit volcanic feelings of the past and produce complicated problems. Staff of hospitals and institutions for the elderly have increasingly noted more severe reactions in this group of patients and their families than usually observed among other Jewish aged.

Feelings of intense anxiety and depression, even dreams and

nightmares of Holocaust content may erupt in confrontation with diagnostic procedures, surgery and confinement. During the Holocaust, health took on a particular significance and disease meant an automatic death sentence. This awesome feeling may still persist.

Even the common phenomena of old age, such as reduced activity and mobility, or impaired hearing and sight may bring back unresolved feelings of powerlessness and doom, at times experienced as a sense of "I did not escape."

While such reactions are definitely not common to all survivors, they are known to occur and need to be understood within the context of the historic past. In such situations, it is important to help the survivor separate the "now" and the "then" and cut short the process of retraumatization. Expressions of empathy, ventilation of the tormenting emotions, brief exploration of the Holocaust incidents, and other psychological supports may help in preventing a chronic fusion between these different traumas and these different frames of time.

Sense of Guilt

Survivors of the Holocaust often manifest a strong sense of guilt. This may reemerge with potency at times of crisis, particularly around loss of family or friends. Again, this seeming overreaction can be understood as a legacy of the genocide. Many survivors had witnessed the destruction of their entire family and community and have truly survived the collapse of their world.

Experiences of such massive trauma can never be fully confronted or "worked through." The expression of mourning and reinvolvement with some aspects of life that gives "meaning" may serve to reduce the duration and intensity of this phenomenon called "survival guilt."

Sense of Family

Family is a loaded concept for survivors because of the total or near total destruction of all members. In working with this population we need to be familiar with the currently proliferating literature on the subject. These writings overwhelmingly confirm the existence of unique bonds in Holocaust families. Children have been often perceived by survivor-parents as the meaning for survival and the reason to be. In turn, the second generation is known to have experienced intensive conflict in breaking away because of guilt in imposing pain on parents who had suffered such cruel and multiple separations.[17]

No wonder that illness, institutionalization or death of an aging parent may elicit in the son and daughter, now adult, a set of complicated grief reactions that are related to the ever present issues of loss and mourning that binds and transcends generations of Holocaust victims.

Absence of Kin

Aged survivors without kin may be a group at risk and may need strong community supports, including outreach. These individuals are truly alone in the world, since the earlier surrogate families of fellow-survivors are now also gone. A social worker who provides services to this population noted that most are unable to fill in the question regarding ''next of kin'' on the agency's application blank.

Diversity of Survivors

Holocaust Survivors are not a homogenous group. Therefore, community services and programs must consider the diversified backgrounds and different life styles.

Need to "Bear Witness"

Holocaust survivors have a strong need to "bear witness." As eye witnesses to this unbelievable chapter in human history, survivors want to make sure that the Holocaust not be forgotten and that future generations know about it in ways that are not distorted. They bemoan the frequent efforts of the media to commercialize, popularize, trivialize and inappropriately universalize the Holocaust. Their rage, however, is unending when confronted with lies spread by revisionist historians who try to "prove" the Holocaust never existed or that its gruesome aspects are an exaggeration.

In the face of such outrageous efforts to rewrite history or to deny the facts, survivors are bursting with an urge, as never before, to speak out and set the record straight. Aware of their advancing age and decreasing life expectancy, survivors are particularly eager to speak out *now*.

There are poignant manifestations of this strong need—individual and collective—to "bear witness." This has been demonstrated in the recent world-gatherings of thousands of Survivors in Jerusalem (1982) and in Washington (1983); in the extensive commemoration activities organized by survivor groups; in the massive outpouring of oral histories, and other testimonies. These memoirs often include reminiscences about their families and communities before the Holocaust and thus offer invaluable, authentic knowledge about a world that was totally destroyed by the Nazis in their war against the Jews.

According to Erikson[18] and others, life review is an important task in the final cycle of human existence as it brings the needed reconciliation with the past and acceptance of one's life as it has been. Given the nature and intensity of survivor guilt and the incomprehensibility of the Holocaust events themselves, it is questionable that life review serves a similar function for the aged Holocaust survivor.

Instead, the readiness to publicly evoke the hellish memories may represent the never ending need to commemorate the dead, to speak for those who were silenced and to tell the world what genocide is about and what are the ominous signs to predict it. These processes and objectives are intertwined, as evidenced in the public mass gatherings of survivors which combine the private act of mourning with the act of evoking public conscience about the events and lessons of the Holocaust.[19]

In working with aging Holocaust survivors and perhaps victims of other mass destructions these needs must be understood and harnessed creatively for they may help in restoring a meaning to survival and may mercifully promote an integration of brutally fragmented lives.

REFERENCES

1. Conot, Robert E., *Justice at Nurenberg* (New York: Harper and Row, 1983).
2. Bush, address on Capitol Hill, April 1983.
3. Deborah Lipstadt, *Shoah*, Vol. 1, #4.
4. Report to the President, *President's Commission on the Holocaust,* Superintendent of Documents, U.S. Government Printing Office, Washington, D.C., 20402.
   Dawidowicz, Lucy, *War Against the Jews: 1933-1945.* (New York: Holt, Rinehart, Winston, 1975).
5. Baron, Salo, "From a Historian's Notebook: European Jewry Before and After Hitler" in *Out of the Whirlwind,* ed. Albert H. Friedlander (New York: Doubleday, 1968), pp. 133-54.
   Celia Heller, *On the Edge of Destruction* (New York: Columbia University Press, 1977).

6. Rosenbloom, Maria, "Experiences in Survival Outside the Concentration Camp" (paper presented at "Conference on Social Work Practice with Holocaust Survivors and Their Families" co-sponsored by Brookdale Center for Aging; Self-Help, Inc.; and Hunter College School of Social Work, New York, 1979.)

7. Frankel, Victor, *Man's Search for Meaning* (New York: Simon & Schuster, 1964). Wiesel, Eli, *Night* (New York: Avon Books, 1958).

Levi, Primo, *Survival in Auschwitz: The Nazi Assault on Humanity* (New York: Collier Books, McMillan Co., Inc., 1958).

Wander, Fred, *The Seventh Well* (International Publishers, 1977).

Goldstein, Bernard, *The Stars Bear Witness* (New York: Viking, 1949).

Ringelblum, Emanuel, *Notes from the Warsaw Ghetto* (New York: McGraw Hill, 1958).

Winick, Myron, *Hunger Disease* (John Wiley & Sons, 1979).

8. Bettelheim, Bruno, *The Informed Heart* (Glencoe, Illinois: Free Press, 1960). Levi, *Survival in Auschwitz*. op cit.

9. Frankel, *Man's Search for Meaning*. op. cit.

10. Dimsdale, Joel E., *Survivors, Victims and Perpetrators* (New York: Hemisphere Publishing, 1980), p. 240.

11. Donat, Alexander, *The Holocaust Kingdom* (New York: Holt, Rinehart & Winston, 1965).

12. Krystal, Henry and Niederland, Willing, *Massive Psychic Trauma* (New York: International University Press, 1968).

Bettelheim, B. *Surviving* (New York: Alfred Knopf, 1979), pp. 28-37.

13. American Psychiatric Association, Task Force on Nomenclature and Statistics. *Diagnostic and Statistical Manual of Mental Disorders*, 3rd Edition (Washington, D.C.: American Psychiatric Association, 1980).

Figley, Charles R. *Stress Disorders Among Vietnam Veterans. . .* (New York: Brunner, Mazel, 1978.)

14. Bettelheim, *Surviving*.

15. Daum, Menachem and Rosenbloom, Maria, "The Meaning of Survivorship in Late Life Mental Health," grant application to National Institute of Mental Health (New York: Hunter College, Brookdale Center for Aging and The School of Social Work, 1982).

16. Lifton, Robert Jay, "Observations of Hiroshima Survivors" in *Massive Psychic Trauma*, ed. Krystal, p. 174.

17. Epstein, Helen, *Children of the Holocaust* (New York: G. P. Putnam's Sons, 1979.)

Fogelman, Eva, "Therapeutic Groups for Children of Holocaust Survivors," *International Journal of Group Psychotherapy* 29 (April 1979), 211-235.

Bergman, M. and Jucovy, M. *Generations of the Holocaust* (New York, Basic Books, 1982), pp. 83-102.

Linzer, N. *The Nature of Man in Judaism and Social Work*, Federation of Jewish Philanthropies, New York, Chapter on "The Social Worker and Survivors."

Solkoff, N. "Children of Survivors of the Nazi Holocaust," *American Journal of Orthopsychiatry*, 43:3, 1974.

18. Erikson, Eric, R. *Childhood and Society* (New York: Norton, 1950).

19. Kaminsky, Marc, "Survivors' Stories: From Private Nightmare to Public Action," presented at Conference, *Survival Stories*, Hunter College, Brookdale Center on Aging, June 2 and 3, 1983, New York City.

Section IV

*PERSPECTIVES FROM
THE WORLD OF PRACTICE:
EMERGING SOCIAL WORK
APPROACHES AND SETTINGS*

Chapter XIII

The Senior Center:
Informality in the Social Work Function

Sondra M. Brandler

INTRODUCTION

The new students have arrived at the senior center with the appropriate mix of anxiety and eagerness and the usual questioning about the assignment and the placement. This field internship is hardly what they expected social work to be. The workers are dressed in casual clothes, few ever sit at their desks, and lengthy conversations with clients are conducted between the office and the restrooms. Those clients or workers who seem to be engaged in structured activities are listening to music together, drawing pictures, or cha-chaing around the dining hall. Many are playing games. Something about all of this is bizarre. Where is the therapy about which students are supposed to learn? Did they come to social work school to teach baking? Everyone is on a first name basis, and lack of rank and station in this circus make it difficult to identify the performers. Even the field instructor, who at the moment is assisting in tying a shoelace for an elderly participant, seems more like a social director than a social worker. The students are confused, some not overly enthusiastic about working with older people in the first place and others disappointed in the population for not being dilapidated enough, not demonstrating their neediness. If these older people are so able, what purpose is there for a fresh-faced student interested in helping? Some students want clinical work and cannot imagine that this carnival of a center is capable of offering training for them. It appears on the surface that counselling, marital work, family therapy are not possible here. In general, for students and other less interested people, looks can be deceiving.

The senior center is an eccentric social service agency, unique in its costumes, sometimes unconventional in its approach. The informality of the setting often leads the newcomer to believe that nothing of great importance is happening. The recreational element, the fun, creates in the best centers an atmosphere which belies the seriousness of the purpose. If the center is to be effective in reaching out to older people, whether at a time of psychosocial crisis or during the more routine course of daily events, it must be a place which radiates a sense of comfort, warmth and familiarity, which invites but does not intrude. People perceiving only the atmosphere have misconceptions about the nature of the agency.

To achieve the real goals of the center, the special needs of older people in meeting the challenges of aging must be recognized and a program designed with those needs in mind. The blending of needs with activities is subtle, not easily discernible to every new student. Key also is the role of the professional worker in providing support to clients while encouraging them to maximize independence. Here, too, the process is a delicate one and is best understood over time. Students must learn that through a program which stimulates emotional, intellectual and social growth, the senior center becomes a conduit for developing creativity, mastery, and a renewed sense of self for many older participants. The therapy, which in other settings is meted out in formal sessions, evolves in the senior center.

The consumer, participant or client, the program, and the worker are the center. How these three intertwine forms the fabric of the center and makes each center pattern somewhat different from others. Nevertheless there are commonalities. Basic themes emerge, themes which connect to the aging process and to its relationship with center life. By examining the three elements, who is being served, what vehicle is being used, and what is the role for a professional worker in the setting, one can begin to understand the significant contribution to community social services which the senior center can offer.

THE CONSUMER

Harry, long retired, whose wife is much younger and still employed, struggles to feel useful and potent. Mary, in charge of "twenty-five girls and a million dollar budget" until her heart attack and forced retirement, searches for new directions for her energies. Dora, with a history of depression, needs to talk with peers and to find an outlet for her considerable talents as a writer. Some have found that eating alone is intolerable. Others want to discuss the news. Some always wanted to dance, to paint, to sing. Still others are leaders with no one to lead, bakers with no one to savor their pastries, craftsmen with no one to admire their work. The majority of center participants are in their seventies, are retired and are in relatively good health. They are experienced, capable and fairly vigorous, with the exception of some frail elderly in specialized programs, and they represent a range of socioeconomic statuses consistent with the range in the aged population as a whole.

The handlebar mustache is the distinctive feature, the crew cut, the plaid shirts, the quality that is somehow larger than life. Jack is a man of loud laughter, exaggeration, bravado and stories about growing up under the stars in Montana. Those who know him well say that the tales are more bluster than truth, that Jack spent his early life on the Lower East Side of Manhattan and has some remote association with the West but never actually lived there. It seems irrelevant. The fantasies capture the sense of the man, Jack who is powerful, who fancies himself a cowboy or, at the very least, an outdoorsman, Jack, who is full of vitality and who claims he hasn't visited a doctor since he had his army physical in World War II.

These are the facts. Jack worked as a lineman for Con Edison until his retirement in 1978. He is 71 years old, married, the father of four, the grandfather of three. In 1977, Sarah, Jack's wife, who is also 71 years old, suffered the first of a series of major strokes which left her left side paralyzed and her speech distorted. She is now able to walk but moves with difficulty. Jack went from king of the hill to permanent nursemaid. He cajoled, encouraged, prodded Sarah to make efforts to walk and talk, and, in many ways, he is credited with her progress. He did and continues to do cooking, housecleaning and shopping which Sarah is unable to manage. It is Jack who has nursed Sarah, looked after her personal care, worked with the doctors and therapists. As Jack explains it today, doctors describe Sarah's current condition as a "time bomb." Travel, to which both Jack and Sarah had looked forward, is impossible. Nearly all activities are restricted.

After more than one long hospitalization and after several critical points in her illness, Sarah came home to a life devoid of interest, with little opportunity for socialization, and no relief from the imprisonment of her mind and body. Jack, too, was chained to home. The daily routine centered on meals, trips to the doctor, television watching and sleeping. In nice weather Jack varied the schedule by taking Sarah outside to sit in the sun for a few hours, but inevitably they returned to the same routine. Those who remember him then say that it appeared that a part of Jack, the noisy part, the buoyant part, was irretrievably lost.

In June of 1979, a senior center opened two blocks from Jack and Sarah's home, and a neighbor suggested that Jack and Sarah might like to join. Jack volunteered to go with the idea that the center might need some help in getting started, help that he could provide. It was easier to think of himself in the helping role rather than as a center participant, and help he did. Despite her disabilities, Sarah too was put to work. She prepared table settings for the lunch program, a job she could handle while sitting and one that could be managed with only one hand, and she supervised the registration table.

It has been five years since Jack and Sarah first came to the Center. Today, the two can be seen every morning at 8:00 A.M. or earlier getting the Center in order for the other members. Jack keeps the inventory, arranges for trips, cleans the building and does other odd jobs. He holds the keys, opens and closes the building. Most important, Jack serves as dining room manager, seeing that all two hundred or so daily participants are greeted, seated and fed. He and Sarah rarely eat in the center themselves (Jack is too busy, and Sarah must be on a special diet). Jack is a foreman of sorts, or so he sees himself, and both are thriving.

Jack and Sarah are special, but their story is typical of thousands of others who have found their way from loneliness and inactivity to socialization and enrichment at the senior center. Utilization of the senior center relates in no way whatsoever to psychopathology and unlike other services to the aged is not called into play only when problems present themselves. Nonetheless, in the course of "normal" aging there are various psychosocial issues which must be confronted, and for many participants, the senior center can be thought of as a therapeutic community in which to deal with these issues. Adjustment to retirement, to illness, to widowhood, and to a myriad of possible social, economic and emotional crises often precipitates the decision to join a senior center. For some consumers, who may have come to the center with only a casual or passing interest in some of the trips or activities, crises are faced at a later date, and involvement in the center provides continuity and support in times of trouble. Relationships fostered in the center carry over to other hours, and an active center participant is likely to have friends to accompany her to the movies, to visit her when she is ill, and to grieve with her when she suffers a loss.

There are those who use the senior center only occasionally when they need assistance or information related to concrete problems—housing complaints, entitlements, or homemaker services, for example. Having found a receptive atmosphere in which to discuss these issues, many return when they have other kinds of concerns. One man attended a center once a year when he needed assistance with renewing his senior rent exemption. During these visits, he would tell the worker about his difficulties in sharing his home with his older sister, and the simple application procedure would turn into an hour-long discussion. Four years after this process began, the worker received a telephone call from a hospital. The man had died, and his last comments to his sister were to instruct the hospital to call the center in her behalf. The center, in effect, had become her next of kin.

Not all center participants are persons one considers as socially active. There are those who do not appear to be searching for more intimate relationships. Some involve themselves in no center activity, speak little, eat their lunches and return home. They utilize the center as an indoor park, a place where it is acceptable to be a quiet observer, alone yet in the company of others. This level of involvement is sufficient for them. Others seem to desire more but have difficulty in taking the initial steps. The reticence of some participants needs to be overcome, the energy of others demands direction, the skills of many await discovery.

THE PROGRAM

An awareness of the needs of the center population should shape the program, and these needs will vary according to region, ethnicity and economic status of the participants. Common to all program designs, however, must be several underlying themes which relate the program to certain life tasks of aging. These life tasks fall into two major categories, adjustment to loss and adaptation to change. The intrapsychic conflicts, the self-esteem issues, the family problems, the socialization difficulties which afflict all of us are intensified by the struggles of aging, and although the importance of the recreational element in programming should not be underestimated, recognition of the relationship between activity and psychosocial well-being is essential.

The program of the senior center should be responsive to the losses experienced by older people. The groups must offer, in both concrete and less tangible manners, ways of working through feelings of depression, isolation and impotence and, at the same time, ways of improving socialization skills. Although some groups appear to be recreational or educational in nature, all groups should be therapeutically oriented. An example of this is the senior center baking group. It suffices to justify the formation of the baking group on the grounds that persons in the center enjoy baking, but a well-designed center program takes more into account.

Ten women and two men have signed up for the group. The men are professional bakers and the women baked in their own homes in years past. Nine of the group members are widowed, live alone and have no one for whom to bake. Several are on restricted diets and cannot eat the baked goods themselves. The group starts amid a flurry of organizational problems, not the least of which is how twelve people can work together in one kitchen amicably and efficiently. No one of the twelve is willing to volunteer to do the shopping, and three women regularly get the cleanup detail. There are many ongoing arguments, yet most of the group members continue to attend. In the course of group meetings, the meaning the group holds for members becomes apparent. Nearly every session is replete with stories associating one particularly marvelous chocolate cake recipe with a special past event. Each woman tells of a time when the party was in her home, when she cooked and baked for an army of appreciative guests. All the associations between feeding and family surface during the conversation, the joys, the regrets, the memories. The men are admired as the professionals and get some opportunity to demonstrate their skills for the others. The pride in past accomplishments carries over to the present. Reminiscence can be a powerful tool in ego strengthening, but the baking group has the additional virtue of providing the older person with a measure of current accomplishment. When the cookies come out of the oven and a crowd of customers gathers, the aromas of cookies and success intermingle. No greater compliment could be offered the bakers than the opportunity to sell their goods, earn some money for their center and rave reviews for themselves. The group bakes for immediate sale or for the use of the center in holiday and birthday celebrations, and group members know that they have made a contribution to center life. The bakers also have developed a special camaraderie, and a few have made friends in the group. The organizational difficulties will never be fully resolved and crop up anew as the group composition changes. Nevertheless, group members work out some system of taking turns in choosing the recipe, supervising, and doing the chores.

The therapeutic value of the baking group will depend in part on the way in which the worker handles his/her role. There are various approaches, but all must be oriented to the real purpose of the activity, which is to respond to the needs of group members in adjusting to loss and in finding meaningful roles. The baking group is a nearly perfect activity for its members, because the activity is in itself pleasurable and satisfying, the response of customers is positive and, consequently, supportive, and the opportunity for self-expression and reminiscence, is continuous. Although they enjoy baking, these older people would have little pleasure from it if they baked at home and had no one to appreciate their products and no one with whom to share the experience. Old age is a period of continuing emotional and intellectual growth, and programs should reflect that growth. The process of systematizing a way to divide the tasks in baking a cake develops socialization skills and, in turn, promotes that growth. In addition to giving an emotional boost to members, the sale of the baked goods and the provision of cakes and cookies for party refreshments actually benefit the center. This activity is recreational, therapeutic, educational, social, and it encourages group and center participation.

In planning this or any other activity, goals must be thoroughly explored. A similar activity or even the same activity might be designed with a different purpose. For example, the men's cooking-for-one group, although it also deals with food preparation, is quite different in intent from the baking group. While there must be an emphasis on loss, since the men in the group are all recent widowers and discussions often center on the adjustment process, there is also the focus on coping by acquiring skills, by adapting to change. The content of the activity, learning to cook nutritious, well-balanced, economical and tasty meals, is important to survival for these men. They must be able to care properly for themselves alone, but many are totally unprepared to do this. The goal of this group, without denigrating the importance for the men in having a chance to express themselves, to offer friendship and support to each other, is for the group participants to learn to cook.

The senior center program should meet the social, psychological, intellectual and physical needs of participants. Activities, always with a therapeutic base, fall loosely into several categories: those chiefly of an educational nature, those that are recreational, those designed to promote social action, those to encourage creative pursuits, those to provide physical exercise, those to promote voluntarism, and those to deal with emotional difficulties. Each activity may be age-specific or not. Educational programs, for example, might be varied to include lectures on nutrition, drug usage, hypertension, and senior tenants' rights. They might also include book discussions, sociology classes, music appreciation, and science programs. Again, the underlying importance of the activity must be understood: Educational programs, in providing information, help participants to cope better as older persons in a changing world. Additionally, learning gives a person a sense of control, mastery and potency, which contributes to psychological health.

Recreational activities can be utilized to achieve center goals, although professionals sometimes undervalue their importance. Card playing, while fun, is mentally stimulating and provides socialization. Other games challenge coordination, increase skills, encourage learning. Outings and trips, which would be impossible for some older people to participate in without the community of the center and the provision of transportation and organization, give pleasure and enrichment. Movies are more entertaining and holidays and birthdays more festive when they are shared with others. Whatever recreation is offered at the center, the value of the activity is greatly enhanced by the participation of the older people in the planning, organization and execution of the program. In this way, the services seem to be more responsive to what the consumers want, and older adults, who may have felt cut off from control over their own lives, are empowered.

What is accomplished by urging center participants to take part in their own program planning carries over into other areas. Older people vote, but until recently they did not see themselves as a special interest group with political clout. The social action group of the senior center serves a dual purpose by allowing its members to feel useful, vital and strong and by supporting causes which will benefit all older people.

Many older people who prior to retirement had neither the time nor the inclination to pursue certain interests join groups which encourage creativity. The center becomes the showcase for formerly undiscovered talents, providing the structure and the incentive for the development of expertise. Some people paint for the first time, and others compose poetry or appear in plays. Knitting, ceramics, photography, singing, crafts, sewing, woodworking, and writing are just some of the group activities which fill the center calendar. With groups of this sort, as with all other center activities, the goal of the program must be clear: to provide self-esteem through achievement and to inspire self-expression and creativity.

Many senior centers have recently introduced into their programs physical fitness activities, which are quite popular with center participants. Classes in yoga, exercise and aerobics, in various forms of dance and in several different sports provide participants with a sense of well-being and cultivate social interaction. A favorite activity in one center is belly dancing. An outing to a Mid-Eastern restaurant, featuring a professional belly dancer, capped off an exciting season for this class. Participants, vigorous in mind and body, feel alive and attractive. People with disabilities can and should be included in exercise and dance programs, if these programs are modified appropriately.

For some older people, the only way to continue to affirm purpose in life is to have a work role. Although they offer no salary, volunteer jobs replace former roles and give meaning, structure and satisfaction to numbers of older people. The senior center, by encouraging participants to take an active part in the government, organization and daily operation of the center, provides opportunities for older persons to feel useful and needed. This is a somewhat complicated situation, for the volunteers who run the center are both workers and clients. Although no financial remuneration is provided for them, there is some tacit expectation of tangible reward in terms of volunteer recognition and sometimes in terms of access to service, which may be construed by other participants as favoritism. Volunteer groups in the senior center must include an ongoing training component and careful supervision to assure that while the participant has the opportunity to volunteer, s/he is performing the tasks capably and fairly.

In addition to the contribution that the volunteers can make to the center itself, there are roles for volunteers in service to the community. Some centers arrange for their volunteers to assist at hospitals, schools or libraries. In other centers, volunteers design toys or knit articles for distribution in hospitals or other institutions. What this means to the volunteers might best be illustrated by the story of Anne, a seventy-four year old woman in a volunteer sewing group at a senior center. Anne has difficulties in getting along with other people. She is easily offended and given to outbursts of temper. Acquaintances at the center describe Anne as suspicious and irritable, someone who is hard to know and harder to like. Anne has had a troubled life. She was widowed at a young age, raised her only child alone, and when her son was eighteen years old, he was killed in an accident. Anne lives alone and has no close family or friends. The volunteer sewing group which Anne joined at the center was formed to make specialized apron-size bibs for developmentally disabled wheelchair patients in a local facility. The bibs are made from white towelling and are cut and hemmed with bias tape by the volunteers. The job is boring, but the companionship of the group and the knowledge that the work is to help the handicapped eases the tedium. Anne thought that decorating the bib might make the individual using it feel that it was a more personal gift, and she began to embroider designs on each bib and match them to the color of the tape on the hem. Bright boats, balloons, flowers, rainbows and clowns adorned Anne's bibs, and her idea stimulated others to try to create their own pictures. Anne became a leader of the group with others asking for her approval of their designs and requesting her assistance. After a few months, the volunteer sewers took a field trip to the facility utilizing the bibs and were delighted to see that their bibs were being used and were especially appreciated by the residents. Since those who had embroidered certain bibs could recognize their own designs, they felt a bond between themselves and the user. The group spoke about the visit to the facility for months afterwards and has since returned there on several occasions. Anne has made friends in the group and feels less alone. It has given her a sense of belonging and direction.

Any senior center activity, by virtue of the fact that people have the chance to socialize, learn and enjoy together, can be therapeutic. Some issues, however, require more direct action. Groups which deal with the crises of aging, the widows' group, the caregivers' group, the stroke patients' group, are essential to the senior center program. Also important are groups, like one billed as a psychology of aging discussion group, which address, in a general context, concerns of older people. A typical session might deal with sexuality or depression or intergenerational conflict. Groups of this sort may be open to all center participants or may be limited by invitation only. As in any other therapeutic setting, workers in the senior center can determine those most appropriate to the group. If it seems desirable, the worker may also elect to use some vehicle to engage group participants. The film discussion group, the reminiscence group, the poetry therapy group, the men's club may in reality have the same focus as the psychology of aging group or the widows' group. The inclusion of these kinds of groups and the approach which assures that all center groups are oriented to therapeutic goals distinguish the professionally led center from other centers.

THE SOCIAL WORK ROLE

The social worker in the senior center plays many parts. In some centers, she/he is responsible for everything from maintenance to budget, from meal planning to policymaking, performing all the traditional roles, and standing in lieu of family for some center participants. All tasks relate to two basic objectives, to provide older people with needed support and to assure that older people maximize independence. These are the major concerns of the social worker whether as administrator, as group worker or as caseworker. The objectives must be achieved with a consciousness of the group interests as well as those of the individual.

The Social Worker as Administrator

The social worker administrator in the senior center has a peculiar balancing act to perform. On the one hand, s/he must necessarily divest herself/himself of authority and power in order to allow participants to make their own decisions, to be in control and to feel able. On the other hand, the worker must make the professional judgments which define the setting as a therapeutic one for all participants. The complexity of this balancing role is more easily understood in terms of an illustration from practice. A volunteer, who has given a great deal of service to the center and who is in charge of the daily sign in for participants, has had repeated arguments with one older man. The nature of the disagreement is unclear, but ugly words have been exchanged between the two men, and during the latest argument, the volunteer announced loudly in the company of others that he will see to it that the man is expelled from the center. The administrator is aware that to permit the man to continue to attend undermines the volunteer. To ban attendance on the grounds that the participant has insulted the volunteer is not an acceptable solution. The choice of who may use the center and who may not can become a kind of popularity contest. The difficult social work task is to assure the volunteer of his status and importance to the center while not expelling any participant. Maybe the individual whose behavior is the most upsetting to others requires the service the most. Helping that person to become integrated into the center and to act in a socially acceptable manner is beneficial to both the individual and the group.

Even decisions which are arrived at in a democratic fashion are not necessarily in the best interests of the group, although these decisions do not have the arbitrary flavor of the volunteer denying services to a troublesome participant. The members of the trip committee may schedule an outing which they believe that some people would enjoy. Since the committee as a governing body is something of an elite and its planning reflects the committee members' interests and ability to pay, outings may be arranged which are too costly for many participants. The social worker must guide the committee and interpret for committee members the needs of the community of the center.

While some activities should be offered in the senior center program which have broad appeal, others which provide a service to a select group are also necessary. The acceptance by a senior government, as part of its center program, of a class for foreign-speaking older people to learn English can be a major source of conflict. When centers have attempted to introduce blind older people or frail older people into their programs and have offered special services to these groups, other participants have balked at the idea. Here too the social work administrator is responsible for deciding what services to offer and to whom. The process of educating senior advisory boards to the needs, recognizing and exploring their concerns, serving as a role model, working with the indigenous leadership in a cooperative fashion, effectively training volunteers and enlisting their assistance, is the multifaceted and difficult task of the social work administrator. She/he must accomplish all of this while maintaining an atmosphere in the center which is warm, friendly and inviting. Even the tone set by the administrator in handling complaints about the size and color of the apples on the dinner tray becomes important in creating that atmosphere.

The Social Worker in Work With Groups

A primary responsibility for the social worker in the senior center is as a worker with groups. The earlier discussion of senior center programming suggests some of the content of group discussions, both latent and manifest. It also suggests some of the theoretical considerations in establishing particular groups in the senior center. The professional group worker in all settings is concerned with group formation, development, and problem-solving, with improving communication and socialization skills, but there are differences between group work in the senior center and in other types of facilities. In the senior center, some group sessions relate to aging, all participation is entirely voluntary, and participants may elect to participate in numbers of different groups while attending daily. With these factors in mind, the group worker has the formidable challenge of keeping groups fresh, interesting and varied.

It is usually impossible for every group to be conducted by a professional social worker, impossible because of limitations in staffing, time and money. Many groups have been organized to learn particular skills, and group leaders must be expert in the appropriate discipline even if they are not always sensitive to the underlying center goals. More often than not, a key responsibility of the social worker is to provide supervision to group leaders who are not social workers. These leaders may include older participants with skills in other areas. Sometimes the decision may be made that a particular individual would benefit from the opportunity of becoming a group leader and may be well suited to the task. A highlight of the week at one senior center is the current events discussion led by a center participant and his wife. The two conduct the sessions as if they were on a radio talk show, and the good-natured banter, not exactly the stuff of traditional group work, is enjoyed by all.

Since many activities in the center are primarily educational and since participants come from a background of respect for authority, they tend to have an image of the group worker as teacher. Added to this is the notion bought by many older people that aging has made them powerless and incompetent and that they have little to offer. As such, group members often are reluctant to take any responsibility for the group, are wary of contributing their thoughts since their opinions may not be the correct ones, and expect that the worker will be expert in the subject area. Group members in a literature discussion group, for example, may be fearful of choosing the story to read and discuss, will not volunteer to take a turn at reading aloud, may arrange their seats in rows and are likely to raise their hands and await recognition before speaking. After the story is read, all eyes center on the worker who is expected to provide an explication. The group worker must facilitate group discussion in a way which will assure that the focus shifts back to the group. It is helpful for the worker to consider that she/he is a facilitator rather than a group leader, that true leadership rests with the participants.

The group work role in the senior center is further complicated when one considers the responsibility generally held by the authority figure for discipline. If a group member is disruptive, if she comes into the session late and disturbs the discussion, or if she insists on speaking on her own agenda when the group is intent on something else, then participants look to the worker to mete out punishment. If she/he assumes the role of police officer, the worker confirms the belief that group members are incapable of protecting their own interests, that old people are weak and helpless, and she/he infantilizes the disruptive group member. A better approach involves assisting the group to create a contract which can be appealed to in various situations. With the issue of lateness, for example, the group might elect to lock the door at a certain time and not admit latecomers. This is a group decision which the group executes. The contract is constantly evolving, and one role for the worker is to help members to apply it as necessary in establishing the limits for the group. If a participant cannot be helped to control her behavior in the group, she probably has some problem that needs further intervention either on an individual basis or in another kind of group. Group members understand that the participant whose behavior is unacceptable to the group cannot be barred from attending, and the worker can help the group to handle disruptive behavior through discussion. The worker models more effective ways of dealing with inappropriate behavior, tries to channel comments that are long-winded or irrelevant to the topic, makes the connections between participants, interprets and mirrors. The entire process should be directed toward empowerment of group members and improving social interaction for all participants.

The Social Work Role With Individuals

Unlike utilization of a mental health clinic, attendance at a senior center is not stigmatizing. Older people who are participating in activities, socializing, or eating lunch are comfortable in the center and often less threatened than in other settings in approaching the worker to discuss a problem. It is not unusual for someone whom the worker knows only casually to ask to talk about some personal issue. Neither is it uncommon for the worker to greet someone in the hallway only to find that the chance meeting develops into a lengthy discussion. Those who are alone need someone in whom to confide, someone who listens and is empathic and supportive. Flexibility and informality are required of the worker, and it is sometimes difficult for the worker to differentiate between her roles as friendly companion and as trained professional. Most often individuals who ask to speak with the worker come with concrete problems—the Medicaid card has not arrived, a form needs to be filled out, there is a leak in the apartment. The social worker must have the information and know how and when to refer a matter elsewhere, in short how to negotiate the system. Above all, the worker must be aware that clients in the center are capable of doing much for themselves and, whenever possible, should, with support, be handling their own affairs. Helping the older person to see how much he can do for himself is good practice.

One tricky part of the process is understanding that a simple request for assistance in interpreting a form may be the presenting problem but not the real issue at all. As in any setting, the social worker must be alert to verbal and nonverbal cues as to what is really happening with a client, but since the center is not thought of as a traditional mental health setting, more pretext may cloud the issues. Many requests for help come about because older people feel inadequate or depressed. Some experience a nonspecific malaise, a feeling that they have no energy to address the daily life crises, and they come for help around a concrete concern because they are unable to identify the larger problem.

Some information about the functioning of a center participant is available at intake if the intake worker is attuned to the hidden messages. An older volunteer can be trained to be cognizant of certain signs which suggest that the professional should get involved. The participant is asked who she would like to notify in case of emergency, and she gives the name of a funeral home; the participant is asked whether she is taking any prescribed drugs, and she lists numbers of medications including antidepressants; the participant is asked for the telephone number of a relative, and she replies that her son refuses to give her his new telephone number. Intake interviews in which the newcomer seems confused, depressed or suspicious are interviews which need follow-up. Also requiring follow-up are interviews which take an excessive amount of time because the participant needs to talk. In short, the social worker, by being alert, can with minimal information identify the client in trouble. Most people find their own way into the center community, but with knowledge of the special needs and difficulties of some participants, the social worker can ease their integration into center life.

The role of the social worker in the senior center, whether it is related to administration, work with groups or work with individuals, is to give a sense of strength, meaning and joy to center participants. Ideally, center participation should be broadening, should encourage spiritual, emotional and intellectual productivity and health. One participant, in a letter to the social worker in her senior center, sums it up by writing, "You gave me a reason to wake up in the morning. Thank you."

ADDITIONAL READING

Butler, Robert and Lewis, Myrna. Aging and Mental Health. St. Louis: Mosby, 1974.
Einstein, Gertrude. "What Does Life Mean To Us Now That We Are No Longer Young?: A Series of Group Discussions at the Southwest Seniors' Hospitality Center," Social Work With Groups, Vol. 3, No. 2, Summer, 1980, pp. 65-74.
Kaminsky, Marc. What's Inside You It Shines Out of You. New York: Horizon Press, 1974.
Kubie, Susan H. and Landau, Gertrude. Group Work With The Aged. New York: International Universities Press, Inc., 1953.
Meyerhoff, Barbara. Number Our Days. New York: E. P. Dutton, 1979.
Pincus, Allen. "Reminiscence in Aging and Its Implications for Social Work," Social Work, 1970, 15 (3), pp.47-53.

Chapter XIV

The Use of Aged Volunteers: Individual and Organizational Considerations

Robert Salmon

The volunteer in social welfare has a long and rich history. Up to the turn of this century and before social work was organized and recognized as a profession, volunteers were the primary advocates for service to the poor, the old and sick. These individuals performed essential work as advocates as well as providers of services to those in need, and clearly fulfilled the role definition of a volunteer, described in a current dictionary as "one who offers himself for service of his own free will."

However, in 1956, the volunteer in social agencies was defined as ". . . a person who, without financial compensation, supplements the work of paid staff."[1] This definition infers the organizational locus of the volunteer's efforts, and specifies the adjunct relationship to paid staff. It is possible in the specificity of this definition, to see the genesis of the often negative, or ambivalent reactions to the volunteer in social agencies. The *Encyclopedia of Social Work*[2] has reported that employed social workers often are unsympathetic to volunteerism. They have not been sufficiently trained to work with volunteers and as a result, they make inadequate and ineffective use of them. It has been said that the concern about "Issues such as professionalization, role delineation, confidentiality, volunteer dependability, and volunteer supervision . . . " as well as ". . . Social Work's preoccupation with psychotherapy and confidentiality, have limited volunteer activity of and participation in the practice of social work."[3]

This is a revised version of an earlier article by the author, "The Older Volunteer: Personal and Organizational Considerations," *Journal of Gerontological Social Work*. Fall, 1979.

Often, there are political or economic concerns about the use of volunteers. The National Organization of Women expressed their view:

> Women who take volunteer positions as part of an underpaid work force in organizations perpetuate the economic inequity of women in the work place. Volunteers and other workers who are paid less than a living wage, thus obscure the true value of their work. They are not compensated according to their contribution either by status, job security or money.[4]

In speaking about the older volunteer, it has been said that:

> . . . voluntarism must supplement and not be a substitute for what should be a gainfully employed work force. It is obvious that until we have an economy and social system that dependably provide and insure job and career opportunities for all those of preretirement ages who want and need employment, tension will exist between the laudable goals of retiree volunteerism and the reality of an insufficient number of jobs at decent wages.[5]

An even stronger position was that:

> We are unalterably opposed to any programs that exploit older people by asking them to perform, on a voluntary basis, community service work for which younger people would receive a nominal wage. If the older person has the skills to perform such work satisfactorily, and the service being provided is one needed by the community, then the community should be willing to pay for it.[6]

Another factor to be noted is that "citizen participation and volunteerism has been a steadily decreasing force in the public welfare structure . . . The client population is among the neediest, often the least "attractive"; clients frequently live in very isolated places or in crowded slum areas considered "dangerous," or at the least unsavory, by middle class volunteers."[7]

The age of the older volunteer adds another dimension of concern specifically related to our attitudes about older people. Agency executives and workers are subject to the same preconceived, stereotyped view of the aged as the rest of the population. Their anxiety about using older volunteers may be expressed in organizational terms; it may take too much time; the volunteer may be ineffective. They may feel that ill health of the 70 to 80 year old may interfere, and attendance may be irregular. In these times of budget cuts in particular, agency executives and their professional staff are over-burdened, and they may view the volunteer as an additional work assignment in a job already difficult to perform. In these rather human terms, they may resist the idea and actuality of a volunteer program.

> Since agency executives must be concerned first about the sur-vival needs of the agency, and of the potential a volunteer pro-gram may promise the agency, it is quite appropriate for an ex-ecutive to want to know what "is in it" for the agency. I would maintain, as a good many others have before me, that individ-ual older people and agencies can benefit considerably from volunteer programs. In order to achieve a level of success in attracting volunteers, however, a primary emphasis has to be on the needs, interests, and differences of the older people the program seems to attract, and then of the needs of the agen-cies.[8]

Clearly, both are important, and will be discussed in this chapter.

The increasing literature of the aged, as well as of that of the older volunteer,[9] is but one indication of the growing importance of the aged in this century. Their problems have increased as their numbers have grown. Poor health, poor housing, limited employ-ment possibilities, and low income are often associated with increas-ing age. All of this has been substantiated[10] and publicized.

Another kind of problem also has been cited in the literature. It concerns the loss of an established role, when retirement begins.

> With job and family responsibilities at an end, it is the rare aged person who can claim a place for himself which he, his peers and younger persons alike regard with respect. No longer the breadwinner, or the acknowledged head of the fami-ly, the average elderly individual has lost the role that he understands and the community respects. It is difficult for him to maintain his former self-image and the community offers him little help in doing so.[11]

The loss of previously held and valued roles is difficult for individuals of any age, and perhaps it is felt particularly keenly by the elderly. Volunteerism can be a source of satisfaction for the elderly and a tangible way to create a functional and status bearing role for the elderly. "Those people who view retirement as a source of potential fulfillment and believe they have something valuable to contribute are those who respond most positively to the work of the (volunteer) project."[12] Conversely, many view retirement as a time of problems and conflict. Therefore, the task of creating this role is a difficult one. We have been conditioned, in our society, to obtain primary satisfaction and status from instrumental values—those associated with one's employment or household role—but status bearing roles for older people tend to stress expressive values—those associated with service, socializing or recreation.[13]

Volunteerism may serve to meet this problem by offering service to others, an expressive value, through instrumental tasks already familiar to the volunteer in other forms. In order to do this effectively, ". . . the volunteer jobs must have specific hours and specific length or terms of commitment. . . . preset terms of commitment . . . allow the older volunteer to work and contribute within a staff structure without feeling he is embarking on another twenty year career."[14] It also would help if we were able to provide volunteer programs that fully consider the differences of the older people we seek to attract.[15] Old people do have certain shared characteristics—they have lived long enough to be and look old. However, as is so in any age group, they have attitudes, experience, habits and hopes that differ markedly. Agency staff who develop programs while considering the aged as a sort of homogenized entity make a serious mistake. An environment for work, for service, in which the volunteer feels useful, valued and productive is one in which individual differences are considered and utilized.

> . . . Volunteer loss or turnover is a problem . . . factors causing senior volunteers to discontinue their participation reflect their feeling of dissatisfaction. . . . if older volunteers are not esteemed or valued, no matter how responsible the tasks, they will have low job satisfaction.[16]

The agency role in this is crucial. Gratification must be provided and pain avoided if the agency is to attract and retain volunteers. Stanley Levin, in discussing the importance of the work setting, emphasized the creation of an atmosphere that:

—Emphasizes the importance of the older volunteer.
—Facilitates the satisfaction of the older volunteer's expectations.
—Reflects sincere care about older volunteers and genuine appreciation of their satisfactory performances.
—Extends opportunities for maximum application of the older volunteer's skills and experience.
—Provides avenues for the older volunteer's growth and development.
—Encourages active participation of the older volunteer in program planning, implementation and evaluation.
—Offers older volunteers meaningful roles and assignments.[17]

The atmosphere, the conditions for work, are important elements in creating the environment of the older volunteer's assignment. They have to be considered as one develops guidelines for the planning and implementation of successful volunteer programs. This was done masterfully by Sainer and Zanger, out of the SERVE experience, and they identified eight broad guidelines to attract and retain the desired types of volunteers. They are as pertinent now as when they were first developed in 1971.[18]

1. Opportunities to serve that are appropriate to the experience and background of the volunteers must be developed: Often, the placements offered by agencies may be inappropriate for volunteers, and flexibility and innovation may be needed to find opportunities suited for the older volunteer. More opportunities for volunteers can be made available than usually are considered. If they are located, it will be of benefit to the volunteer, and the agency's interests will be served as well.
2. Volunteers should be recruited and trained on a group basis so that the volunteer has a peer group as a point of reference and a source of identity: Through the opportunity to serve, the individual old person will have the opportunity for association and friendship with peers. Many people, including old ones, believe that more can be done by a common effort rather than an individual effort. The fact that many are involved gives the individual a degree of comfort and a feeling of self-worth.
3. Volunteers should be offered a variety of placement choices in both direct and indirect service capacities: Most people are used to working hard at tasks, often concrete ones, in a relatively structured work situation where attendance is expected and regular. If there is a variety of tasks available at different

levels of skill, options and choices are available. This can lead to comfort and a kind of job security, since this comes about when there is regular work to be done, and the volunteer is the one chosen to do it. There is another factor to be considered. Old age is a time, often, of diminishing choices for the individual, in many areas of his existence. We need to recognize this, and as a result, try to give the older volunteer choices in his contact with ourselves and our agencies.

4. There should be no elaborate schedule of pre-training.[19] Instead, orientation should be provided at the agency in the actual service setting: Elaborate pre-training might imply that the volunteer is being tested for fitness, particularly to the volunteer from a lower socioeconomic status. A general orientation, such as individual screening and a work assignment in which the volunteer has as much choice as possible, is helpful. A more specific orientation to the job assignment takes place shortly, when he begins the actual task of volunteering. In this way, the volunteer need not worry about whether he is qualified to do the job.

5. Agency staff should give personalized attention to the volunteer. Absences should be followed up and complaints listened to: Individualized attention, facilitated by a weekly group meeting or group structured program when possible, will help the volunteer move into the agency and promote communication and better relations and understanding with the agency staff.

6. Efforts should be made to gain public recognition from the larger community for the services of the volunteers: All people need reaffirmation of their own worth, and individuals from lower socio-economic status may need even more reassurance. Recognition and praise from staff, friends, officials, and the media is a kind of community sanction. This kind of community recognition and status is a form of important remuneration as it may represent the value society places on the services he renders. It may lead to positive satisfactions and motivated performance. Another form of recognition is through certification. For instance, an increasing number of schools of social work offer continuing education program and/or post-master's certificate programs. There is a great interest in these programs and certificates as they are tangible evidence, not only that the person has completed a specified

number of hours of course work, but that the improved quality of skills has been accredited. If agencies are interested in working jointly with educational institutions to develop certificate programs for volunteers, I believe that the agencies would find eager and willing partners.

7. Transportation and lunch should be provided so that rendering service does not cost the volunteer anything: This is an important factor in recruitment and retention of volunteers. If a group of volunteers are involved, the availability of a taxi, car, or bus from the agency is helpful.

8. No potential volunteer should be turned away because he lacks social or job skills: The experience of those who work extensively with volunteers indicates that some of those who appeared least promising have developed into the best volunteers. Involvement of this sort has provided a means of individual growth.

Sainer and Zanger suggest that their guidelines apply to volunteers of higher socioeconomic status, as well. This is useful to know since it has been reported that "... (older people) with greater personal resources rather than those with greater needs are in a better position to take advantage of whatever benefits a program provides."[20] This kind of volunteer may be more self-directed, able to work without seeing immediate results, and may be able to function in a more autonomous fashion. Some programs are designed specifically to attract this kind of volunteer.[21] Rather than a new direction in the use of volunteers, they may represent a continuation of a long-standing pattern of unequal opportunities to volunteer of the powerless, the poor, and the consumers of service in our society.[22]

However, regardless of their socioeconomic status, volunteers tend to be uninterested in engaging in busy work. The worker gains a sense of achievement when the relationship between what he does, and the objectives of the organization in which he works, are clear and direct.[23] All of us including old people, obtain gratification when our efforts are understood to be useful as well as needed. Although the research on the benefits of the volunteer role to the aged volunteer have not produced consistently positive results, we tend to make an assumption and hold the belief that volunteers will accept positions, benefit from them, and stay with them if their individual psychological growth needs are satisfied.[24]

Up to this point, the discussion has been concerned with work and literature emphasizing the primacy of the needs, interests, and differences of older people if they are to be attracted and retained as volunteers. However, "The *work* itself brings together the interest of the volunteers and the organization. To be meaningful, the work must do two things: induce the volunteers' psychological development and help to accomplish the central goals of the organization."[25]

In order to accomplish this last point referred to by Sequin, the organizational needs of our agencies in relation to volunteer programs should be considered. Agency administrators are impelled to consider them if they are to make intelligent decisions. The organizational factors will be discussed here, drawing extensively and primarily from the work of Sheldon Tobin, and his associates Stephen Davidson and Ann Sack.[26]

Sometimes the use of volunteers will save money for an agency. Sometimes agency executives say that a carefully mounted volunteer program will be of considerable monetary cost to the agency, but it is worthwhile when social work objectives and the benefit to individuals are considered. In fact, volunteers can make significant and sometimes unique contributions to agency life that go well beyond monetary considerations. Volunteers need to be deployed with care as their use is appropriate in some situations and quite inappropriate in others. Considerable research shows the volunteer can be as regular in attendance as the paid worker.[27] Therefore, since volunteers and paid staff can share the same characteristics in this area, there is a need to focus on the distinct organizational differences of paid staff as opposed to volunteers that help to determine the appropriate uses of each in the agency or institution. This needs to be done by comparison.

PAID STAFF

"Two main factors which make the utilization of paid staff attractive are:

—the organization can maintain closer control over the activities of paid employees; and
—the needs of the volunteer might conflict with organizational and clients needs."[28]

An individual who works in one of our agencies or institutions fills a specific role in the agency. He has a job title and a defined place in the organization. The lines of accountability are clear, and the paid worker is expected to carry out his defined tasks and duties. The agency can exercise considerable control over his activities as a result. With a volunteer, however, the lines of accountability may not be as clear. Is the volunteer responsible for example, to a Director of Volunteers, or the Branch Director, or to the Senior Division Head? Often, the lines of responsibility and accountability are not as clear, which makes it harder for the agency to maintain control over the activities of the volunteers. The power of the paycheck is an important factor in this. Even if the paid worker has major areas of dissatisfaction in his work, or disagreements with the authorities, he will tend to comply if he wishes to keep his job. A volunteer receives no paycheck. His remuneration, his reward, comes from the gratification inherent in the task he performs, his feeling of being needed and wanted, and of making a useful contribution as he perceives it, to clients and the agency. It is possible to conceive of situations where a volunteer's rewards, such as feeling needed by clients, may get in the way of important moves towards independence by these clients. Since employees receive paychecks, it may be more possible for them to give up this particular reward than it is for the volunteer.

VOLUNTEERS

"Three characteristics of volunteer staff suggest ways in which they can best be utilized. Volunteers make useful contributions to the agency, the community, and individuals because they:

—Are more knowledgeable about the community;
—Can function as advocates; and
—May enhance the client's sense of competence and worth."[29]

Many volunteers come from the local community in which the agency is situated. Frequently, the paid workers do not come from this local community. Therefore, it often occurs that the volunteer will know more about his community and have more knowledge about community resources and the formal and informal helping network than will a new paid staff member. In this situation, the volunteer is a resource to the agency, and may be an important linkage to the community.[30] Volunteers sometimes come from elite groups in the community and may have entry to the local political powers. Volunteers frequently can function as advocates. "Volunteers, both professional as experts, and non-professionals as representatives of the target group, are well suited for advocacy activities because they can promote what appears most sensible for the elderly rather than what is most advantageous for the agencies or organizations."[31] Also, volunteers who are happy with their agency often become the most vocal protagonists for the agency, and this, clearly, is of benefit to the agency.

Much of the literature about older volunteers emphasizes the gratification and feelings of self-worth that may be achieved by the volunteer. However, the converse of this is the sense of well-being and worth they may help elderly clients achieve. Shore describes the basis for this kind of contribution.

> The residents feel that the employees are paid for their affection, and that family is duty bound, but the volunteer comes because she wants to. She doesn't have to come, and this is what makes her really unique . . . Even if the home has unlimited funds (and no home has) the services and the role of the volunteer could not be replaced with money.[32]

Therefore, the client's feelings of self-worth may increase because of this gift of self on the part of the volunteer. "Through the direct services rendered and the psychological benefits imparted, the volunteers meet both overt and covert needs of his/her clients."[33]

It is clear that volunteers can be an asset to the operation of the agency. As indicated above, "for many tasks, they (the volunteer) will be more effective than professionals, providing a more personalized and informal quality."[34] Volunteers should not be used as unpaid staff members to cover budgetary problems. Rather, paid staff and volunteers each have important roles—and roles that should be seen as distinct and separate—in the delivery of services to the aged.

As indicated earlier, one important service is to the aged volunteer himself. It is important "to move in the direction of using more aged staff for . . . our programs. The commonality of life experience among the aged . . . and aged staff can be an invaluable asset."[35] It is important not only for the benefits to the recipients of service, but for the giver. The isolation and sense of marginality experienced by many aged people inhibits the fulfillment of some basic needs. Just as we need to eat regularly, and to take care of our physical needs, we need to meet regularly and repeatedly with friends, colleagues, and others to meet our social needs. The volunteer, in his work, has this opportunity to be a role model for other aged people. Volunteer work, for the giver, may very well decrease the sense of alienation and anxiety that afflicts so many of the elderly. This in itself may be a factor in deferring early institutionalization for some of our old people.

The combination of clear and long-range benefits to the aged volunteer and to the recipients of his services, and the potential organizational benefits to agencies, all add up to powerful arguments for the creative development and implementation of volunteer programs. In these difficult times, when the needs of our older people, and of the social agencies that serve them, are often neglected or denied, the importance of this task is clear.

REFERENCES

1. *Volunteers in Selected Casework Programs: Standards for Their Use*, Community Council of Greater New York, June 1956, p. 1.

2. Seider, Violet and Kirschbaum, Doris. "Volunteers," *Encyclopedia of Social Work*, Volume II, N.A.S.W., Washington, D.C., 1977, p. 1583.

3. Schwartz, Florence. *Voluntarism and Social Work Practice*. A report on a project funded by The Lois and Samuel Silberman Fund, New York, September 1981, Appendices pp. 7, 8.

4. National Organization of Women. *Volunteerism: What It's All About*, 1973.

5. Gotbaum, Victor and Barr, Elinor. "On Volunteerism." *Social Policy*, November/December 1976, p. 51.

6. Hutton, William "Volunteering: Unaffordable Luxury for the Elderly." *Generations*, Summer 1981, p. 13.

7. Guyler, Catheryn and Halberstein, Gloria. *United States Government Memorandum: Regional Survey of Volunteerism in the Delivery of Human Services*, January 20, 1982, pp. 9, 10.

8. Salmon, Robert. "The Older Volunteer: Personal and Organizational Considerations." *Journal of Gerontological Social Work*, Fall, 1979, p. 69.

9. For instance, see *Volunteers in Human Services* (Human Services Bibliography Series), Project SHARE, November 1980. This publication of the Department of Health and Human Services is an annotated bibliography of literature relevant to the effective use of volunteers in human service organizations. A number of the publications that have been annotated are concerned specifically with the older volunteer.

10. Op. Cit., Hutton, p. 12. The author cited figures from the United States Bureau of The Census that 400,000 more older individuals, in 1979, were added to the below poverty level income group, the largest increase for older Americans in twenty years. Fifteen percent of those 65 or older were in that group. With inflation increasing substantially since then, the figure is higher now.

11. Sainer, Janet and Zanger, Mary. *SERVE: Older Volunteers in Community Services,*

A New Role and a New Resource, Community Service Society of New York, 1971, p. 1.

12. Stone, Janet and Velmans, Edith. "Retirees as Volunteers: Evaluation of Their Attitudes and Outlook." *Volunteer Administration*, Winter, 1980-1981, p. 6.

13. Sainer, Janet and Zanger, Mary. "Critical Factors in Successful Involvement of Older Persons as Community Volunteers." Paper presented at the 25th Annual Meeting, Gerontological Society, Puerto Rico, December, 1972.

14. MacLeod, Tom. "The Effective Use of the Retired Volunteer." *Volunteer Administration*, Spring 1980, p. 16.

15. This was the approach used in SERVE (Serve and Enrich Retirement by Volunteer Experience) and described in detail by Sainer and Zanger who will be cited frequently in this paper. SERVE was the model for the Retired Senior Volunteer Program (RSVP) which is a Federally aided program in existence in many parts of the country.

16. Rakocy, Genevieve. "Senior Volunteers: Funding and Keeping Them," *Generations*, Summer 1981, p. 36.

17. Levin, Stanley. *Volunteers in Rehabilitation*, Goodwill Industries. Washington, D.C., 1978.

18. Sainer, Janet and Zanger, Mary. "Guidelines for Older Person Volunteers." *The Gerontologist*, Autumn, 1971, pp. 203, 204.

19. Sainer and Zanger's point that there should be no elaborate schedule of pre-training may not always be appropriate in light of the circumstances that exist in 1982. Seider and Kirschbaum, op.cit., p. 1590, commented that neither NASW nor the Council on Social Work Education had given serious attention to volunteers. That situation is changing. On September 17, 1982, in a letter to Hunter College School of Social Work, and other schools, Dr. Arthur Katz, Executive Director of CSWE announced the application for funds in order to conduct a national demonstration and training project to prepare older persons for volunteer work in human service agencies. The key element in the proposal is training. In the Description of Volunteer Training Program, it was stated that, "By preparing a trained volunteer labor force of senior citizens, human service agencies will enhance their service rendering capabilities while providing appropriate volunteer opportunities which tap the potential contributions of older persons."

20. Kornblum, Seymour. *The Meaning of a Volunteer Role to the Aged*. Research Digest published by the Florence G. Heller Research Center, New York, 1979, p. 34.

21. For example, see *Older Volunteers Program in Hospitals*, The Hospital Research and Educational Trust, Chicago, Illinois, 1981, p. 4 and Stone and Velman, op. cit., p. 4.

22. Seider and Kirschbaum, op.cit., p. 1583.

23. Sequin, Mary and O'Brien, Beatrice. *Releasing the Potential of Older Volunteers*. The Ethel Percy Andrus Gerontology Center, Los Angeles, University of Southern California Press, 1976, p. 53.

24. It should be noted that this assumption, and belief is not always validated in the limited number of research studies that have been conducted on the effect of a volunteer service role. Kornblum studied the impact of the volunteer service role upon the aged participant in the Jewish Ys and Centers of Greater Philadelphia. He said, "The major purpose of this study was to determine the effect of a volunteer service role on the health, morale, self-perception, social interaction, and level of activity of participants in the RSVP program. We found that participation in the RSVP program had no effect." (Kornblum, op.cit., p. 29). Charles Fogelman's study produced different results. (See Fogelman, Charles, "Being a Volunteer: Some Effects on Older People." *Generations*, Summer 1981, pp. 24,25.) He studied a group of older Americans who had been volunteering in the federally sponsored Senior Companion Program. He found, in part, that volunteers are better off socially, emotionally and physically than those who are not volunteering; they were less lonely, and believe their help to be vital. The conditions and circumstances of these studies cannot be elaborated on here. However, it is fair to say that the actual impact of volunteer roles upon the aged individual has not been thoroughly researched. Kornblum pointed out that most of the research with this group has been concerned with predictors of successful retention, and the factors that effect retention. (Kornblum, op.cit., p. 2)

25. Sequin, Mary. "Social Work Practice with Senior Adult Volunteers in Organizations Run by Paid Personnel." *Journal of Voluntary Action Research,* April - September, 1982, p. 55.

26. Tobin, Sheldon, Davidson, Stephen and Sack, Ann. *Models In Effective Service Delivery: Social Services for Older Americans.* Submitted to the Administration on Aging, H.E.W., The University of Chicago, School of Social Service Administration, January 1976.

27. See, for example, Faulkner, A.O. "The Black Aged as Good Neighbors: An Experiment in Volunteer Services." *The Gerontologist,* 1975, Vol. 15.

28. Op.Cit., Tobin et al., p. 110.

29. Ibid., p. 112.

30. For elaboration, see Litwak, Eugene, "Community Participation in Bureaucratic Organization: Principles and Strategies." *Interchange,* Vol. 1, No. 4, 1970.

31. Op.Cit., Tobin et al., p. 113.

32. Shore, H. *Adventures in Group Living.* Dallas, Texas, Golden Acres Home, 1972, p. 211.

33. Op.Cit., Tobin et al., p. 114.

34. Schwartz, Florence. "The Professional Staff and the Direct Service Volunteer: Issues and Problems." *Journal of Jewish Communal Service,* December, 1977, p. 148.

35. Salmon, Robert. "The Group Experience for the Aged of Today." *Journal of Jewish Communal Service,* Spring, 1970, p. 253.

Chapter XV

The Arts and Social Work: Writing and Reminiscing in Old Age: Voices From Within the Process

Marc Kaminsky

Poetry, Coleridge said, brings the whole soul of the poet into activity. That's a way of putting it. Wallace Stevens repealed the *soul* and repeated the dictum for our modern ears: "Poetry is part of the process of the poet's personality." Writing, a writer would say, "feels like everything"—part of the world with which one makes contact; part of the self in its moments of wholeness, a feeling and a means of integration. For a writer, writing is a generative, a creative act: the word becomes flesh—not an artifact, but a living thing. Whitman's "Leaves of Grass," for instance, are the poems on the page; his innermost, departing thoughts ("the frailest leaves of me"), as he stands before us for the thousandth time, saying good-bye; his fragrant physicality ("the scented herbiage of my breast"); the green surface of the earth, which is a sacrament, being "God's handkerchief"; the title of the book he worked on all his life; his fate, as it is everyone's fate, for Whitman was continually aware that "all flesh is grass." Perhaps more boldly than anyone before or since, he confessed what poets feel when he said, not in these words, "Take this book; it is my body."

Critics may "deconstruct" the presence of the writer, so that they can possess the pure body of the text; they may deflate the imagination which bestows being on syllables. But no poem could be written, no art made, without faith in a resurrection, in a "second life of art": Eugenio Montale's faith that the value of a work of art lies in its unpredictable and "obscure pilgrimage through the conscience and memory of men, its entire flowing back into the very life from

225

which art itself took its first nourishment . . . A fragment of music or poetry, a page, a picture begins to live in the act of their creation but they complete their existence when they circulate . . . Paradoxically, one could say that (they) begin to be understood when they are presented, but they do not truly live if they lack the capacity to continue to exercise their powers beyond that moment, freeing themselves, mirroring themselves in that particular situation of life which made them possible. To enjoy a work of art or its moment, in short, is to discover it outside its context; only in that instant does the circle of understanding close and art becomes one with life as all the romantics dreamed.''

For a writer, the letter giveth life; periods of not writing are little deaths. And so when a person of Coleridge's faith—and Whitman's and Stevens' and Montale's and that of any true poet—enters the workshop, he may never need to teach the most fundamental thing that he has to impart: his feeling that writing is a life-giving act. It is in the atmosphere that he carries around him; it is a kind of spiritual axiom upon which the development of talent depends. And isn't it natural that the faith of such a person would have special value for people whose old age comes in an age of shattered faiths?

Writing, for a writer, is not therapy: it is life. And a vision of life; in our century, a violent, death-haunted vision. ''The important thing,'' said Camus, ''is not to be cured, but to live with one's afflictions.'' By writing the writer bears what he knows and sees and suffers and is. There is no cure. We live in the century that reveals its character most by its inventiveness in terrorizing and murdering vast populations. Existence, as in other dark times, feels precarious. For us, art is no longer a refuge. Poets may go on seeing beauty, as before, but it is likely to be the sort of ''terrible beauty'' that Yeats found in ''Easter, 1916.'' Rilke, in the first lines of the *Duino Elegies*, discovers that ''beauty is nothing but the beginning of terror we're still just able to bear.'' James Wright, watching a high school football game, sees American boys grow ''suicidally beautiful'' as they ''gallop terribly against each other's bodies.'' Those old people whom we account wise know that the intensity of life we yearn for may arise out of self-destructiveness, and that no good can come of denying paradox, chance, and evil. They know there is no cure: we're imperfect, we're guilty, and we die. And they welcome a vision of things adequate to their knowledge.

If they distrust poetry, it is because they have been taught that poetry shows us nothing but the land of our heart's desire. But the imagination constructs its pleasure domes or Sunday mornings, its open roads or Byzantiums so that it may have a place apart, on which to stand, beyond the reach of "the average expectable environment"; and there it looks out upon things as they are and sees what cannot be seen if one doesn't have what Virginia Woolf called "a station in midair." The imagination is not to be dismissed because it is a light and floating thing: without it, poets couldn't rise above narrow circumstances and reconnoiter the real.

The writer, upon entering the workshop, hopes to teach people to write as writers do: out of the pressure of life upon the imagination, out of necessity. It is useful, even pleasurable, to teach grammar, prosody, the secret paths of metaphor; but it is necessary to bring the whole soul into activity.

And this takes time, and repeated attempts to capture a feeling or a peculiar slant of light that lies just beyond the reach of the words we've learned to deploy. Six or ten sessions won't do it. But given time—say a year or two—the writer is able to impart the experience that corresponds to the faith of poets. The people in the workshop come to discover that writing is neither a single activity nor a single process. It comprehends dreaming and observing, spontaneity and calculation, intuition and skill; it elicits, energizes, gives form and direction to the "buzzing, blooming confusion" of thoughts, memories, feelings, and perceptions that pulse through the mind in odd clusters, glimmering for a moment—then they're gone. Writing redeems them. It salvages odd scraps of experience. It transforms receptivity into activity, loneliness into solitude; silence becomes part of a dialogue with a *thou* whose absence or presence awakens new powers of speech.

And the writer listens to what the people in the workshop say. The feelings which their voices manifest enable him to feel meaning in the workshop. Later, their voices return to him, like a musical phrase or a line in a poem that comes back to liberate what is really going on—and marvelous—from its routine appearance. He can no longer talk about the writing workshop without calling on them, for their individual voices have become part of his understanding of what the workshop means. When he arranges their voices into an abstract order, a kind of chorus that sums things up, he hears them affirm that the workshop brings into play a wide range of emotional and intellectual processes that have adaptive value in old age. That's a way of putting it, but their individual voices speak more powerfully, more memorably, than the collective affirmation they make.

Listen! They return to speak about writing, about reminiscing and aging, about being in an art-making workshop; they are saying it enables them:

1. *To continue learning:*

> I was very hesitant in the beginning. School to me—when I was growing up in Germany—was like a military school, discipline and listening. And when we started with grammar here in the group, I really wanted to run away. I was really afraid. I cannot write rhymes, and grammar to learn at this age was for me horrifying. But I must say I learned a lot, and it was not the school type that I thought it would be. It's a very relaxed group, and when I do one bad work the next one is a little better, and I don't feel I'm a failure. In the beginning I was very much afraid I could not go with a group in English. I was afraid of my mistakes, and it all worked out so beautifully that no one cares if I make mistakes. I write what I feel like. I have learned quite a lot.*

—Irene Salamon, Astoria Workshop[1]

> I was asked to join the writing workshop, and I didn't want to. I do love English, but I was upset about the word 'poetry.' I can't rhyme, and I didn't want to start something that I already had a feeling I wouldn't like. However, I became very interested, was also a little argumentative, I'd forgotten that poetry doesn't always have to rhyme. I was completely bewildered by the first poem the writer brought in. I couldn't get anything out of it, and it was English, it was simple, short, and then we took his attitude and so many things came out of every word! He's very analytical, but it's like an injection that you get; they give it to you directly in your blood because it's the fastest way to get to you. It just has to go into your blood, a little goes here, a little goes there, and you hear, see, and then you look at the poem and you understand it; but at the beginning it's nothing,

---

*Quotations followed by an asterisk are from an interview of the Astoria Workshop by Janet Bloom. See "A Window was Opened to Me," *Teachers & Writers Magazine*, 12(1), pp. 12-14.

[1]Four senior centers conducted under the auspices of JASA (the Jewish Association for Services for the Aged) were the sites of the writing workshops whose participants are quoted in this piece.

and that is the way other things are. Once he gave us an assignment about color, and I thought: Now what can I write about color? Now I don't say that every time I wrote something it was what I would have liked to have done, or as well, but I saw something that I didn't see before. And as it came to me, the words, a little window was opened to me. It's hard for me to describe in words. I see a little clearer, I hear a little clearer perhaps, and not only as far as poetry is concerned. As I say, he injected the words, I don't mean it's painful, he opens up a little window, and it's better than no window. Once at three o'clock in the morning, I wrote a poem, a poet I may never be, but I am a little window. It all came to me.

I look at poetry differently now—it's clearer, it's closer to me. I don't know if I can enjoy reading heavy poetry much better than before, but I read it, I feel it differently. It's satisfying. I feel I've learned. It's late in life, but I seem to be able to learn, I think, from every little contact that I have.*

—Aurelia Goldin, Astoria Workshop

2. *To draw upon unused skills, experience, knowledge; to put themselves to use; to make full use of their powers:*

I joined the writing workshop to stimulate my mind once again. I felt that I was stagnating. My other interests were emotionally fulfilling but not necessarily mentally fulfilling. I needed another source of challenge.

—Bea Lipsett, Astoria Workshop

Now that I'm no longer committed to a job, I find it necessary to do something to keep my mind working. As you're growing up, you have to go to school. Then when you get married, you have a family, then you have certain responsibilities. Then when you go to work, you have your family, and your work, and your responsibilities, and sometimes it gets to the point where it feels like it's choking you. And so, when you stop working, and your family is grown, and you don't have to worry about them anymore, then you feel: "Well, gee, now

---

*Quotations followed by an asterisk are from an interview of the Astoria Workshop by Janet Bloom. See "A Window was Opened to Me," *Teachers & Writers Magazine*, 12(1), pp. 12-14.

this is time for me.'' Which is something that you couldn't do
before because if you have an infant it has to be washed and
fed and dressed; as the kids get older you have to take them to
school and bring them back and forth. And so this is the time
of your life when you can say: ''The hell with everything and
everybody, now I can take care of me, and I can do as I please
and the way I please.''
I never liked routine. I always fought against it, even as a
kid. They said. 'You have to eat at twelve o'clock.' If I'm not
hungry at twelve, I didn't want to eat, and this caused problems. But this class, I made it my business to miss as little as
possible, because I really enjoy it very, very much and got a
lot out of it. So this is what happens with most of us—you
become sort of a free spirit that you don't have to worry for
everything, and it's primarily yourself you're taking care of,
body and soul.

—Margaret Friedman, Astoria Workshop

3. *To return to a "road not taken"; to resume an interest of their
youths; to fulfill an abandoned ambition:*

I am interested in the arts, was a millinery designer. I went
to City College night classes, studied sketching and designing;
later on—many years later—I studied Oriental Brush Work at
the Y.M.C.A. And now the greater desire I've had I am fulfilling with this writer's group. I find I now have the ability to
write my thoughts and give vent to my innermost feelings and
to write with confidence.

—Millie Goemann, Rochdale Village Workshop

In *Silences*, Tillie Olsen speaks of those who could not fulfill ''the
greater desire,'' of ''the silence where the lives never came to the
writing. Among these, the mute inglorious Miltons: those whose
waking hours were all struggle for existence; the barely educated;
the illiterate; women. Their silence the silence of centuries as to
how life was, is, for most of humanity.'' The writing workshop
allows their lives ''to come to the writing''; allows us to hear the
testimony of the silent ones: the songs, tales, superstitions, life
wisdom of the furriers, ''operators by blouses,'' survivors of two

world wars, the housewives, ordinary working women, ordinary working men, the many remarkable people among them.

The most important regret I have—but rather I will call it negligence—is that I did not go on to college. While in high school, my plans were to become a teacher and once I was able to take care of myself financially to continue on with the study of journalism. I had always wanted to write and felt by doing it this way I would not have to depend on my parents. But many times, plans do not work out.

I finished high school at the height of the Depression. Conditions were very bad, and I decided to go to work for a while to make it easier for my parents. They urged me to continue with school, we would be able to manage, but no, I wanted to do my share.

Some of my friends, who were in the same situation, decided we ought to do something political in order to help shape a better world. When people were evicted for non-payment of rent, we helped put their belongings back into their apartments. We picketed for people to get what they called "home relief" in those days. Maybe the little we did helped. I like to think so. But all this activity kept me from going back to school.

It still would have been possible but it was neglect on my part and I can only blame myself. It is good for youth to plan and dream because without their dreams and plans some of the wonderful books, works of art and scientific discoveries would not have happened.

—Margaret Friedman

4. *To satisfy their need for continued accomplishment; to create a "finished product" which satisfies their desire for beauty and truth and which has value in their eyes and in the eyes of others; to affirm themselves as creators, makers, workers:*

I wish, I wish, I wish I was a painter and could put on canvas what I see looking through my window. An autumn scene with bare trees, a light dusting of snow on dry grass. A seemingly grim, desolate picture. But as I lift my eyes skyward, I perceive dark gray-black clouds drifting from the northwest with patches of blue here and there. The near setting sun, peeking out now and then, is casting a light pink glow all around the horizon. The red brick massive buildings serve as a contrast to the multicolored panorama. The electric lights look like sparkling ornaments.

One hour later, a complete change of scenery. The electric lights sparkle like jewels while the after-glow of the sunset is a deeper pink with gray topping. I wish, I wish I was a painter and could express my elation and excitement perceiving all this!

—Norman Hofferman, Rochdale Village Workshop

What does a picture of a face mean to you? "Choose a picture of a face and write a poem or story about the face." Within fifteen minutes each of the women in our workshop showed the picture she had chosen and read what she had written.

What imaginations! What a delightful time I had, watching and listening to the enthusiasm the women felt and expressed.

When we were given this assignment, I felt it would be dull and uninteresting, and now I hope I can find the words to do it justice.

Seven women were present at this session. As our writing teacher entered the room, the women were all looking at pictures brought in by Julia Schubert, who told us: 'All my life I wanted to identify with something beautiful. When I was twelve and fourteen years old, I wanted to be an artist. At that time there was a newspaper in circulation called the *Journal American*. A woman artist by the name of Nell Brinkley made drawings of the faces of pretty women, which were printed in the paper. Each day, after school, I sat with that newspaper in front of me and made pencil drawings of some of her faces. Times were hard, there was no money for drawing paper, crayons or paints. My material was the butcher's paper that was used to wrap meat. It had a certain gloss to it that I liked.' And here, many years later, were the drawings on butcher paper! Everyone commented that it was a shame Julia hadn't been able to pursue an artist's career, they were so good.

When the writer looked at the picture and heard Julia's story, he immediately gave us the assignment.

After the last woman read her piece, he said, "Now look again at the picture you chose and write another piece. If you wrote a poem the first time, now write a story, and take a different point of view. If you spoke in the voice of the woman's daughter, now be her sister or her jilted lover. Or is she the one who's been jilted?" We wrote new pieces. Then each of the women, in turn, read her work. Following each piece, we were asked for our comments. The encouragement, empathy, and understanding shown me made me feel it was a joy to be able to do with words what Julia does with lines and shadows.

These pieces were written in a short period of time with no preparation. The ideas expressed and imagination used made me aware that people, like wine, become more flavorful with age.

—Phene Dreher, Astoria Workshop

5. *To communicate with themselves; to explore their inner worlds through writing, through conversing with themselves apart from the presence of an intrusive audience; to turn their loneliness into solitude; to become more aware of their feelings, reveries, dreams; to have an outlet for socially unacceptable feelings of grief, loneliness, frustration, pain, rage:*

Here I am once again. So many things come out of my mind. Tonight I want to write about that. I was just thinking of my late husband. I had a dream about him and he was talking to me just like he was alive. When I wake up, I think: this is only a dream, but it was so real. He told me, "Don't worry too much. I am next to you, and nothing is happening to you," and such a thing comes from the mind. "Go ahead," he told me, "go ahead. You have to live. I am in the next world and it's a beautiful place to stay. Some day you will come, and we will be together."

I accepted that for a while. But my mind is only on him. Maybe some day will come when I won't think too much of this tragedy and my thoughts and my mind will give me a different way to go. Now there is nothing important for me. I refuse to have some time for myself or to go out to a movie or other places. I don't feel in that mood. Of course, in two months it's too early, and I can't forget now this occupies all my time. If I have to do something like shopping, and if I am in a bus or subway, I am thinking of him. No other thing lets me think of other pleasures because my mind and thoughts are only on him.

My children talk to me very often and tell me, "Mommy, you are alive, and you have to keep going." It's the truth. But not for now. Some day I know I want to do things in my way. I love to travel and go places and have good times like other people like to do. I know that will come to me in the future. I don't know when, but I know it will happen for sure if I don't depart soon, and nobody knows when this will happen. I am in God's hands.

Today I was with my son, Charlie. We went to the cemetery to see his grave. The stone has to be put up, and we were going to different places, comparing prices, and everything was very expensive. But for sure I have to put the stone on his grave. There has to be a place next to him in the same place where we have to be together, resting in peace, and forever. This is so sad to say, but it's part of my life, and I have to write all the things that happen in my life, bad and good too. It happens to everybody.

—Margot Rodriguez, East Concourse Workshop

> You think it horrible that lust and rage
> Should dance attention upon my old age;
> They were not such a plague when I was young;
> What else have I to spur me into song?

—Yeats, *"The Spur"*

6. *To communicate with others; to overcome their loneliness by making contact with people who have suffered similar losses, known kindred feelings, struggled with comparable dilemmas; to discover a sense of generational solidarity; to be an active participant in an intimate group:*

I notice because the group is small the people in the group have become quite friendly. It just isn't hello. They really come over and talk. I am not the only one who feels this way. Some of the members of the group say they have opened up more now. I believe that this group has helped many people. It gives you a purpose for coming to the Center and you look forward to it. I believe that most of us live alone and that is why it is important to have a purpose and to be able to express yourself.

—Anne Sager, Astoria Workshop

Self-affirmation should not be thought of as an isolated preoccupation with my individual personality. At just the moment of feeling 'dated' I can realize that others my age feel dated too, and so, in a moment of feeling estranged from my own time, the time-now-past, I discover an unsuspected solidarity, a kinship with others of my own age. They are all peers, my agemates, the people of 'my generation.' They are my beings in a sense that is impossible to escape. Before I even know their names, we share a secret in common. And when we meet and question each other to find a link in our common time-now-past, we already know the link must be there. They are people of my generation, and this kinship is what we share in common. This insight is the discovery of what Ortega Y Gasset calls the 'concept of the generation,' a realization that I belong, unavoidably, to a particular community of human beings who have flourished at a particular time and place.

—Harry Moody, "Reflections on the Living History Project"

To me personally, it opened a whole new world. I could never talk about the past. I opened to it more than I ever thought would be possible, and it feels easy. I can talk in a way I couldn't do even with my own family many times. Yes, here I talk over things I would never have believed it possible to talk about. When I joined the group, I felt I'm the only concentration camp survivor. I felt a patronizing feeling-sorry for me in the group, and I really hated that, but I must say it was all in my mind. Maybe the first few times they wanted to be friendly with me and I didn't accept it, but right now I must say it's the greatest friendship I ever had, and I never had close friends before that I have now. I call them my friends.

—Irene Salamon

Our center is ethnically and racially mixed. This made for strained relationships and subtle hostilities. As a result of the writing workshop, communication has opened, attitudes are changing, and center members have developed greater respect for each other. Racial attitudes have improved—people have found they have common bonds.

—Jane Rosenson, Director, JASA
East Concourse Luncheon Club

It's not only that we write, but we have a chance to discuss. It's drawn most of us out. I mean many times there were topics that we would ordinarily not talk about, but here somehow there is a feeling of real friendship. We don't seem to feel that we have to hold back; we can be really honest with one another. And I think this is a very, very important thing because I have a daughter who seems to feel that people of our generation are not as open with one another as the younger people are today. And with this particular group I find that we do have that open line of communication.

—Margaret Friedman

7. *To become more observant of what is going on in their daily lives, which they often find "empty"; and because they are writing of their immediate world to become more actively interested in the present and to find it enriched:*

Right now I am sitting at my very large window, thankfully not aware of anything in the future. I'm looking at what is going on outside, aware that I'm supposed to be an artist, yet not seeing what is in front of me, not realizing that all around me is beauty. I don't have to look elsewhere. I have a complete view of the sky, bright or gray, the horizon, trees, gardens, and a tremendous plane coming in for a landing, life, people walking, riding bikes, and everything that could enhance the beautiful painting. Yet up till now it was just my window that I have to clean, and I hated it for being so large, therefore saw nothing else. Right now I think: as soon as I'm able to use my arm properly and nothing's cluttering my mind, I will do what I can with what I see now.

—Millie Goemann

Streetcorner Market

Sidewalk fruit and vegetables
Arranged in colorful trays:
Red, purple, green, and yellow,
Each bright color alive:
Nature's paint, an artist's palette.

Fat red-cheeked tomatoes
Look up with laughing puffed faces.
Handfuls of dark red cherries
Send up feelers for tasting
Next to clusters of ripe purple grapes.

Yellow bananas, purple eggplants,
Lemons and oranges, red and green apples,
Lettuce and string beans, all shades of green
Brighten the city around us—
Paris on drab New York streets.

—Israel Raphael, Astoria Workshop

September 17

Right now I am aware of a beautiful Sunday afternoon.
I am aware of the vegetable garden of Rochdale
Village. The Spinach I seeded a week ago already shows
the first green leaves.

Right now I am aware of a grasshopper carrying its
young on his or her back, and right now I am aware that
I never say this before.

—Martha Rosenfelder, Rochdale Village Workshop

8. *To master potentially overwhelming experience; to come into
control of anxieties about failing physical and intellectual capacities; to find meaning in suffering by writing narratives which make a
causal connection between a "bad" experience and a "good" that
came out of it; to order and clarify chaotic feelings in poems; and by
adequate articulation of thoughts and feelings that usually elude or
disorganize the conscious mind, to gain renewed assurance in one's
power to understand, express, and "make" one's own life:*

This morning I woke up thinking about the month of September when I wasn't able to walk. I called up my daughter and asked her to come and see what she could do for me, but she was sick herself. After talking to my daughter, a friend called, and from my voice she asked, "What's wrong? You sound like you've been crying."

I said to her, "I'm so hungry and I can't walk." I had money and food in the house, but could not get to it. In less than an hour, my friend took a cab and was at my house. It took me twenty minutes to get out of bed and crawl to the door, but I made it. She then called my daughter that lives in Jersey. And when she arrived, my friend had cooked enough food to last a couple of days. My daughter from Jersey called my son whom I haven't seen since my brother's death in April, and he came right away. From September up to today, he's at my house every evening with me for a couple of hours. I now cook every day and enjoy a meal with him. I didn't enjoy being sick, but some good came of it.

—Ruth Carter, East Concourse Workshop

I have to fight hard, as I am living alone and my children live far away. I know I cannot be ill, as I will be a burden to my children, and they sure would want to care for me. They have families of their own, and although they have wonderful children, I am sure they have their own problems to solve. I thank God every day as at this writing I am still very alert. I have wonderful children and grandchildren, and to tell you the truth I am living for them, and I cannot afford to be mentally ill at this time.

—Sarah Reiger, East Concourse Workshop

Growing Old

Growing old is like a new shoe that loses its shape from
    too many wearings
Like a new penny that loses its lustre from too many handlings
Or like an old piano that needs tuning up more often

—Lillian Steinberg, Astoria Workshop

Growing Older

People think of me as the Rock of Gibralter,
large, solid, sturdy, and not one to worry about.
I find as I age, although large and solid, pieces
are chipped away. I'm not as sturdy, and hope
someone is worrying about me.

A raging storm makes me think of the youth
I struggled through. Then suddenly the sun peeks
out from under a cloud, and in aging years I settled
down to do the things I wanted to do. I therefore
call these my sunshine years.

The calm sounds of the night remind me of the
late years of my life. Both have the feeling of
serenity, peace, and the knowledge of being.

Getting older has given me a self-assurance
of my capabilities that I never had in youth.

When I am working with clay, it gives me a
feeling of exaltation. In pounding, kneading and
moulding, I'm creating something of earth to which
I shall return.

—Millie Goemann

Growing Old

Growing old to me is a new experience like any other phase of life.
Growing old is like visiting a museum: one admires things of the
    past.
Being old is like an evening after a day of work.
It is like a beautiful sunset on a winter day or a vacation without
    responsibility, a time of leisure.
Being old is like fall time.
Being old is like taking inventory.
Being old is preparing for a long trip to the unknown.

—Martha Rosenfelder

Growing

Growing up is climbing up a ladder to an unknown peak.
Growing old is like reaching the shore after a long and

stormy voyage. You wonder what lies ahead and feel
reluctant to leave the familiar ship.
Growing is a natural process of life. You are expanding
both in body and spirit. It is learning how to live,
and explore the unknown.
Experience is the greatest teacher. If you know that there
is no limit to acquiring knowledge, it can help you grow
young, not old.

—Norman Hofferman

9. *To imagine; to create "lies" that tell the truth; to play with
words, images, ideas, feelings, experiences; to fuse disparate frag-
ments of experience into works that are harmonious, radiant, and
whole; to integrate intuition and knowledge, vision and observation,
past and present, imagination and reality:*

I'm sitting quietly beneath a tall oak tree, listening to the flap-
ping and swooshing and gliding above my head, the rippling
plop-plopping and lapping close by, then suddenly there's a
crunching swirling beneath me, the patter of something approaching. I'm startled, I listen. Nothing. Just "shhh" whis-
tling, and I feel loose, I find myself diddling and daddling.

—Millie Goemann

Refuge

Early morning, I sit on my
            terrace upon the canal.
The sun is rising from the
            east, spreading its
iridescent rays upon the
            calm water.
A boat with its churning
            motor passes slowly by,
making the water swirl
            around. It kicks up the
frightened, fleeing fish.
They find a place of
            refuge, far from harm.
Why, then, can't I?

—Bea Lipsett

In the Garden

The assassin's knife
Plunges into its victim's back
Shedding blood on the roses

—Julia Schubert, Astoria Workshop

Mask

How I wish I could speak
And tell my master the things
He shouldn't do
And the things I wish he would do.

Couldn't he guide me gently
Instead of pulling forcefully on my leash?

When I bark and gaze at him—
If he only returned my gaze
He just might understand that I love and
      obey his every wish.
But he is not sensitive.
I am.

Still I keep on hoping that some day
I may penetrate his feelings, and that
He may in some small measure at least
Reciprocate the love and kindness
      I shower on him.

—Aurelia Goldin

Sounds Like My Life

In 1938 I purchased a beautiful black print taffeta dress that would rustle when I danced. We took the trolley car downtown, the bells went clang, clang, clang as the trolley moved along.

When the airplane was going down, the pain in my ears was such that I wanted to scream.

When I was ten years old, twice, I rode in an ambulance to the hospital.

Now the fire engine passes by at odd hours. Sometimes Lisa, my dog, yodels along with the siren. Napoleon, my other dog, growls if someone is on the other side of the door. I have had six dogs. Each one had his or her own personality. I have loved them all for their silly lovable ways. Each one becomes a part of your life at a different stage of your life: Tootsie, Fritzie, Skippy, Napoleon, and Lisa.

I remember when I was six years old, in West Philadelphia, running after horse-drawn fire engines, and falling down into the sloshing water, getting it in my mouth.

The milkman left the sled, minus the horse, across the street from our house. Everybody rode down the hill on the big sled, but everyone fell on top of me. At another time we played Red Light, a hide-and-go-seek game. I reached the gas lantern first, but someone ran after me and smashed my face into the lantern. Result—cracked front tooth.

Rippling waves around the rowboat made the boat bounce up and down. The lightening flashed all around the house and the trees, making me nervous.

Down in Florida when the sun sets, large bullfrogs come out and make a croaking sound.

—Frances Arluck, Astoria Workshop

10. *To reminisce, to review their lives:*

I like the remembrance of family, and things that happened, and it comes back to you. I love that very much. Memories, and generation gaps, and family, and past and present and future we wrote about, and I love that.*

—Irene Salamon

There's such a—how shall I say?—misconception, and there's such a terribly youth-oriented society that so many people are so afraid: even saying the words "senior citizens" frightens them, as if they don't want to get older. And sometimes I don't think they really know what it's all about because you can get older if you accept the fact that fortunately when you get older you can look back on things in the past and

---

*Quotations followed by an asterisk are from an interview of the Astoria Workshop by Janet Bloom. See "A Window was Opened to Me," *Teachers & Writers Magazine*, 12(1), pp. 12-14.

some of them relate to the present, which is very important and which most of us would not have thought about as much if we hadn't been in the workshop. But here we are made aware of the fact that you can get older and you can do things and you can live a life and be productive and be interesting and be with people.*

—Margaret Friedman

The tendency of the elderly toward self-reflection and reminiscence used to be thought of as indicating a loss of recent memory and therefore a sign of aging. However, in 1961 Robert Butler postulated that reminiscence in the aged was part of a normal life review process brought about by realization of approaching dissolution and death. It is characterized by the progressive return to consciousness of past experiences and particularly the resurgence of unresolved conflicts which can be looked at again and reintegrated. If the reintegration is successful, it can give new meaning to one's life and prepare one for death, by mitigating fear and anxiety. . . In late life, people have a particularly vivid imagination and memory for the past and can recall with sudden and remarkable clarity early life events. There is a renewed ability to free associate and bring up material from the unconscious. Individuals realize that their own personal myth of invulnerability and immortality can no longer be maintained. All of this results in a reassessment of life, which brings depression, acceptance or satisfaction.

—Robert Butler and Myrna Lewis, *Aging & Mental Health*

The memory that is not memory, but the application of a concordance to the Old Testament of the individual (Proust) calls 'voluntary memory.' This is the uniform memory of the intelligence; and it can be relied on to reproduce for our gratified inspection those impressions of the past that were consciously and intelligently formed. It has no interest in the mysterious element of inattention that colors our most com-

---

*Quotations followed by an asterisk are from an interview of the Astoria Workshop by Janet Bloom. See "A Window was Opened to Me," *Teachers & Writers Magazine*, 12(1), pp. 12-14.

monplace experiences. It presents the past in monochrome . . .
Involuntary memory is explosive, 'an immediate, total and
delicious deflagration.' It restores, not merely the past object,
but the Lazarus that it charmed or tortured, not merely Lazarus and the object, but more because less, more because it ab-
stracts the useful, the opportune, the accidental, because in its
flame it has consumed Habit and all its works, and in its bright-
ness revealed what the mock reality of experience can and
never will reveal—the real. But involuntary memory is an
unruly magician and will not be importuned. It chooses its own
time and place for the performance of its miracle. I do not
know how often this miracle recurs in Proust. I think twelve or
thirteen times. But the first—the famous episode of the made-
leine[2] steeped in tea—would justify the assertion that his entire
book is a monument to involuntary memory and the epic of its
action. The whole of Proust's world comes out of a tea-
cup. . . ."

—Samuel Beckett, *Proust*

The phenomenon of life review in old age appears simply as
one form of consciousness—the autobiographical consciousness—which provides the old person with a retrospective version of the meaning of past events—a series of 'metaphors of
self'. . . The criterion of autobiographical truth is to be found
not in science but in art. On these terms, the process of life
review in old age ends in a fictionalized or mythic act of interpretation whereby it is possible to discover—better, create—an
order of intelligibility in one's past, not by remembering it, but
by interpreting it, indeed creating from it new forms of personal meaning.

—Harry Moody, "Reflections on the Living History Project"

11. *To transmit their life experience to those who come after
them, their children and grandchildren; to make socially important
contributions of their knowledge of the past:*

I believe that by recording our experiences, our grandchildren have a way of glancing at the past and they will probably
derive a great deal of pleasure doing that. Also, they may

---

[2]A kind of pastry.

realize that we are more than just meeting for lunch, but getting together in an effort to share our experiences.

We are not old, but simply citizens advanced in the many experiences of life—love, hate, death, life, happiness, all the things that comprise a long life.

—Margot Rodriguez

Writing an autobiography and making a spiritual will are practically the same thing.

—Sholem Aleichem, *The Great Fair*

In their rememberings are their truths. The precise fact or the precise date is of small consequence. This is not a lawyer's brief nor an annotated sociological treatise. It is simply an attempt to get the story of the holocaust known as the Great Depression from an improvised battalion of survivors.

—Studs Terkel, *Hard Times*

Oral history is a record of perceptions, rather than a re-creation of historical events. It can be employed as a factual source only if corroborated. The difficulty of cross-checking information does not detract, however, from its value for understanding perceptions and recovering levels of experience which are not normally available to historians. It offers almost the only feasible route for the retrieval of perceptions and experiences of whole groups of people who did not normally leave a written record. The major contribution of *Akenfield* and *Hard Times* is not their historical accuracy, but rather in their contribution to an understanding of human experience and social conditions.

—Tamara Haraven, "The Search for Generational Memory: Tribal Rites in Industrial Society"

During the last two years of her life, my grandmother worked with me on an oral history of shtetl life and immigration to America "because I want my children and grandchildren should know a little more about the family before us. Zeydeh[3] used to like to talk about the past, he had a lot of

---

[3]Zeydeh: Grandfather (in Yiddish).

memories, but my children weren't too much interested to hear. But it was really interesting what Zeydeh had to say about his past, and little things that I remember from my old country, from my family life with my relatives, in my home. It really should be interesting to my children and my grandchildren where they come from, the roots. Sometimes Zeydeh would remember something, would say something in passing, but they didn't show interest that he should talk more about it. It didn't make him feel good about it because to him it meant something, and to me too. Why shouldn't my kids know where I come from and where Zeydeh comes from and how people lived in his time and the way we were raised and the customs there, and that we also had these things with us and practiced them as much as we would in our life together.''

—Esther Schwartzman

Chapter XVI

The Union Setting:
Working With Retirees

Miriam Habib
Susan Gutwill

The union is a mutual support system which enables its members
to negotiate improved working conditions, wages and a vast array of
benefits such as pensions, medical, dental benefits, credit unions
and, most recently, professional social services.

We will explore the special role of social workers in a union setting, particularly as related to services for the elderly. The program
with which we were involved combined general social work services ranging from counseling and referrals, to group activities and
social action, offered to both working and retired union members
and their families. In this chapter we will describe the program for
the elderly focusing on the special opportunities and problems which
emerged as unique to a labor union setting—an unusual but highly
appropriate setting for gerontological social work practice.

The program for the elderly was directed towards the needs of
two main groups—the active retired seniors and the frail elderly
who were currently or had previously been cared for at home by
their families. The first was called the Retiree Reachout program.
The second, the Caregivers program, was created for the families
(or Natural supports) giving care to their frail elderly relatives. We
will describe each of these programs, emphasizing four major factors which we feel are characteristic of the union setting. Stated
briefly these factors are:

1. A sense of membership and eligibility. Bertha Reynolds, the
first union social worker pointed out the tremendous impact that a
feeling of belonging, a sense that one is a member, and entitlement
have on a client's ability to take help. While everyone finds it hard
to expose vulnerability, working class people find it especially dif-

ficult and feel this difficulty in a particular way. Something wrong is not only felt as painful, but is experienced as a "step down", a failure, a falling into the ranks of the charity cases who are unable to cope or to keep things together.[1] This feeling is not simply subjective but part of the objective experience of lack of respect and appreciation awarded manual workers in this class biased society. For these reasons, it is considered a grave matter indeed to need help and to take it. Everyone who has provided social services within a union format has found that members feel far more entitled to obtain help from their union, which is their own organization than from a nonmembership service agency. Taking help is easier when one pays dues and builds and supports the service which offers help. In addition there is more trust in one's own formal organization or in an informal mutually supportive peer group. The majority of people who came to us for help would not conceive of seeking alternative resources elsewhere. The few that had attempted to do so were actually disappointed in their efforts to obtain help. They felt unheard, unrespected and encumbered by the bureaucracy they could not penetrate. They had often given up in despair and disgust.

Union members would accept services from us that they would reject from elsewhere. Feeling unable to cope and needing help exaggerate the presenting problems and add to the sense of powerlessness of the working class client. At least being a member of the helping organization reduces these feelings of "smallness" a bit.

2. *A sense of working class identity and solidarity.* Secondly, the program was directed towards and sensitive to the special needs and feelings of a working class population. Workers distinguish themselves both from "lower class" people and from more "upper middle class professional and business" people. It was important to understand this sense of themselves and their experiences in order to develop a program which could reach out and hold the members.

3. *A holistic approach.* In this particular program we followed a generic, multifaceted social work model. We related to our clients as union members, as members in need, as group members and as group leaders. Where it was difficult to reach someone in one way, we were able to reach him or her through another aspect of our program. This integrated holistic approach is particularly useful with the union population as they are both participants in program development as well as clients or members in a moment of need.

4. *A host setting with differing value systems.* Fourthly, we had to understand our position as social service professionals within an

organization which was a union, not a professional social service agency. The main goal of the union was to maintain and serve its membership in a time of economic and political decline. To secure trust as we built a social service department and developed programs, we had to be sure that we communicated our commitment to our professional goals as social workers as well as our understanding of the commitment to the union's overall goals. Sometimes these goals differed from each other. The need to obtain open communication in the system was an ongoing task requiring much creative and flexible thinking. There is much for social workers to learn about this aspect of working within a union.

THE RETIREE REACH-OUT PROGRAM

The reach-out program has four major components which developed one from another. Briefly the four stages have been:

1. individual home visits to retired members
2. retiree activity groups in each county
3. a statewide retiree executive board
4. outreach to the homebound retired

The entire service program began with a mandate from union leadership for social workers to join union retirees in visiting other retirees at home. The union wanted to maintain its connection with retirees to ensure their well being and enable retirees to continue contributing to and building the union. Social workers and "retiree visitors," began to make a series of visits. The goals were to establish contact, to assess needs and to ensure that retirees were using all benefits and services to which they were entitled. We found that there were common problems, typical of working class seniors, that were shared by many of the retirees.

The retirees were very often isolated—unaware of community resources and/or afraid or unable to venture out and use them. Firstly many of the retirees did not have access to transportation. Many could not afford a car. During their working years they had managed but now had fewer friends to help and fewer resources of their own. Even if transportation was no problem, many were unfamiliar with community resources which could help them. Even more often, when they did know about available services, they felt uncomfortable and unsure of themselves never having used these services in the past. Restricted to the home, separated from their work lives, often recently displaced from a New York City community to a small town in suburbia, the retirees were all too often unhappy and bored. There were few forces to prevent physical and mental deterioration. The retirees needed the union visits.

Workers work hard, long hours for very little pay and with little flexibility of hours, year after year. They live on the edge of survival. They have little time for the leisurely exploration of their communities. Indeed they are often disinclined to such exploration because they feel unwelcome and uncertain of themselves. Community institutions—schools, hospitals, etc., on their part—do not reach out to, value, or even accurately perceive the experience and needs of the working class. In our experience with the union members they almost always felt anxious in their relationships with institutions and afraid to utilize services and assert their needs and feelings. Sociological literature on the working class family and persons often points out that institutions more often attempt to contain and control working class needs, to help them live with, and adjust to, not question their lives.

As we represented the union we were familiar and welcome where others might be suspect. Retirees felt entitled not only to our help but expected and acknowledged our respect and concern. Above all they hoped and believed that we, the union, would treat them with more sensitivity and respect than they could find elsewhere. We were particularly sensitive to the sense of powerlessness which the retirees felt and recognized that this was often expressed as a reluctance to use resources, medical and social services, even when these were truly needed.[2]

One of the immediate goals of the "visits" was introduction of union and community resources and the education of retirees to their right to these services. We taught how to find and use the appropriate services. For most of the workers with whom we were in contact we were the only helping professionals who had taken the time to help them through their doubts, false starts and hesitations. It was often necessary to escort the retirees to services in their communities and then as they began to grapple with finding a service and using it, we were available to offer support, analysis, encouragement and to advocate directly if needed.

Where many community agencies (we ourselves educated many community agencies to the special needs of the working class and in this process to be more sensitive to their own attitudes toward working class people) have trouble securing volunteers, the visiting program was fortunate in that it snowballed due to the commonality of union membership. A visit made a visitor. Retirees became involved quite easily and were not only interested in participating but thrilled to rediscover old friends and to help again in building the union by helping fellow members.

Quite soon there was a core of visitors and sufficient experience to indicate patterns of problems and concerns. Group meetings were held to describe union benefits and to deal with the common problems and issues. The meeting format was in keeping with the union philosophy of joining together for mutual help and meetings were welcomed as a familiar forum. Participants were honored still to be a part of the union and to remain connected to their past sense of themselves as hardworking, productive people. Naturally not everyone contacted was interested in identifying with the union and some were hostile because of union bureaucracy and politics but by far the greatest response to the invitation to participate was gratitude, excitement and commitment. Members wanted to continue, to meet and socialize and to include retiree group meetings as a regular part of their lives.

It was hoped that these groups would contribute in many ways to maintaining the healthy functioning of the individual retiree. Groups offered a place to go that was familiar and comfortable, counteracting some of the losses of work identity which is frequently part of retirement. Through group participation and especially of leadership development, groups offered retirees a new and important role. The retirees could share with others what they learned about community resources and could themselves participate more in their communities.

From these early "visits" and group meetings, interest has grown, resulting in retiree activity groups in each county and a statewide retiree executive board. The program has become institutionalized.

Fewer members now stay home with nothing to do. A sense of well-being has been maintained and lives have improved. Members have developed speaking skills and feel "good" about the power they possess to win benefits for themselves such as reduced prescription rates, as retirees in the union and the community. Individual horizons have expanded through trips and activities and the adoption of new roles as writers, speakers and group leaders. New friendships have been forged and opportunities offered to affirm the self by reminiscing and sharing special knowledge. The retiree program has maximized the potential for growth in retirement and has shown how much is possible at this stage in life. The program not only prevents deterioration but also builds people and helps them expand and grow. The retirees are continuing their earlier productive role in building the union through the groups and have a means of continuing to interact with working members.

Now that strong countywide groups and a representative statewide retiree body has been established, there is a need to reach out once again. This time it is to the homebound nonactive retiree. To accomplish this task a network of retired members are being trained to make telephone contact and, when necessary, to visit with the retirees. It is anticipated that this reaching out will uncover an increased need for direct service. If this is so, the union, having initiated the program mainly for purposes of information, referral and increased union activity, will be faced with some hard decisions concerning if and how these direct service needs are to be met.

CAREGIVER PROGRAM

The program for those giving full time care to the home bound elderly was another facet of the service for the retirees. In describing it, some of the strengths of the union setting are illuminated. Briefly the program accomplished the following:

1. Helped families obtain direct services.
2. Helped caregiving family members to recognize a need for help for themselves. Caregivers would frequently request help for an elderly parent but not for themselves.
3. Counseled concerning the emotional issues of caregiving.
4. Initiatied a self-help group for caregivers.
5. Facilitated group and union engagement in social action around the problem of caring for the elderly at home.

It is important to understand each of these steps in the program as they relate to the working class population and the union setting.

Many of the members who came with problems of caregiving were not consciously aware of or accepting of the problems they were experiencing. People came to us through a variety of different channels. Usually our first task was to help them become aware of the stress they were feeling as a direct result of their own role as caregivers. One of the first members of our group came to the social workers' attention because she was out of work on disability. After some exploration it became clear that this member was deeply depressed. Although she devotedly cared for her mother, she received nothing but insults from her mother. She developed vertigo, making it impossible for her to "look up at the stairs" at her mother. She could not "go across the street" because she feared her mother's anger and her own feelings of guilt "if something would happen." Another member called because she wanted the retiree program to send her father a birthday card. It turned out she cared full time for two elderly parents—stroke and Parkinson's victims, and both incontinent. One man was referred by his wife who heard of our program at her "shop" and thought we could help "dad." All these people shared one thing: they didn't realize that they needed help and support of their own in the difficult task of caring for the elderly. Unless it was a moment of extreme crisis, our members came for help for someone other than themselves.

If we had not been able to provide multifaceted social work service—obtaining concrete services and making home visits—we would not have reached most of these people, but through our ability to reach out we were able to develop a relationship in which they could begin to explore their feelings as caregivers.

The difficulty that our members had, in defining their own problems as caregivers, was not unique to this population but was exaggerated by the element of class. Caregivers often experience deep guilt, anger and exhaustion. On the one hand people wish their work was over, on the other hand they wish they could do even more. In working class culture where there is less mobility, tighter family units in some ways, more rigidity around sex roles and filial obligations than in other socioeconomic groups, people feel particularly obligated and guilty. Working class people are caught with old values in a new situation and yet have less resources to smooth the edge of the conflicts. There is less money to buy services to ease the burden, there is less of a feeling among workers that they have a right to consider themselves. Workers subscribe more fully than others to the philosophy that one does one's duty, fulfills one's obligations and that one grins and bears it—at all and at any cost.[3]

This heightened sense of responsibility and lack of financial resources was exacerbated in the union retirees by a fear of becoming involved with agencies, services or large institutions which could relieve the burden. Working class people were uncomfortable with the homemaker service, the hospital social worker, the doctor, the nursing home intake worker and the local community mental health agency. Not only ashamed to show and express need, they were also at a loss in dealing with these agencies and thus suffered a double jeopardy. Outside agencies were experienced as confusing, judgemental, evaluators with immense power. Workers felt themselves to be small and inadequate. Much of our role was to teach skills and build confidence to enable the workers to deal with social agencies.

A comparison between the needs and feelings of the union members and those of a middle class client group served by a middle income nursing home, is marked. The middle class client group is assertive and members are able to speak for themselves within the institutional framework because they do have more power and options in this society. In the union setting families constantly need support with asserting themselves and their needs with homemakers, social agencies and organizations.

Several factors contributed to the program's ability to reach members:

1. The existence of a generic program including concrete services, home visits, individual counseling and a group which focused on all the issues and offered peer support.
2. The sense of membership in the union and thus eligibility for the offered services.
3. The recognition by the social workers of the participants as productive workers.

Lastly it is important to discuss the outgrowth of a social action component to the program. As the group developed it became clear that the members were experiencing a problem shared by many others in society. Links were made and other organizations working with caregivers were invited to share experiences. The union members were shocked to learn the statistical proportions of the caregiving situation but were supported to know that others also could feel as guilty, angry and exhausted as themselves.

They were pleased to realise that they could fight for better services and greater awareness of the plight of caregivers through the vehicle of the union. The group joined in a coalition with other groups for better services and distributed a pamphlet throughout the union encouraging outreach to other caregivers. Letters to newspapers and legislators were written. By helping others the retirees helped themselves, for all of this was both personally affirming as well as the catalyst of something useful for others.

CONCLUSION

The two facets of the union services—the retiree reach out and the caregiver program—grew into established programs in a relatively short period of time. Needs existed and the union social service department was able to meet them in a nonthreatening effective manner. Given the perceived distrust of the working class for outside help, it is possible that the union is not only the logical but the key organization which can successfully overcome these barriers with this population. If this is so, unions hold a particular responsibility to act as brokers between retirees and available community services for the elderly and are in a favorable position to provide support to the caregiving families. Benefit to the union is found in continued active membership.

As the aging of the population becomes reflected in an older average age of working union members, and an increasing number of surviving retirees, it is likely that more unions and employee organizations will consider providing services to meet the needs of these retirees and the caregiving family members. The program described here can serve as a beginning blueprint.

REFERENCES

1. Reynolds, Bertha C. *Social Work and Social Living*, N.A.S.W. Publications, Washington, D.C. 1975.
2. Hollingshead, August B. and Redlich, Frederick C., *Social Class and Mental Illness*, John Wiley & Son, 1958.
    Duff, Raymond S. and Hollingshead, August B., *Sickness and Society*, Harper and Row, New York, 1980.
    Sennett, Richard and Cobbs, Johnathan, *Hidden Injuries of Class*, Vintage Books, 1972.
    Stillman, Jeanne M., Davon, Susan, M.D., *Work is Dangerous to Your Health*, Vintage Books, 1973.
    Terkel, Studs, *Working*, Avon Books, New York, 1975.
3. Komorovsky, Mira, *Blue Collar Marriage*, Vintage Books, 1967.
    Levison, Andrew, *The Working Class Majority*, Penguin Books, 1975.
    Rubin, Lillian B., *Worlds of Pain*, Basic Books, Inc., New York, 1976.
    Sidel, Ruth, Urban Survival, *The World of Working Class Women*, Beacon Press, Boston, 1978.

Chapter XVII

Housing for the Frail Elderly: A Model

Roger Baker

It is already clear that the over 75 age group is growing at a rate faster than any other segment of the population. Gerontologists recognized this trend many years ago and began to identify the common characteristics of this subsection and the need for specialized services for it. While no group of individuals can be totally grouped together according to shared characteristics, the over 75 age group tends to exhibit more chronic illness, a greater degree of functional impairment and more frequent episodes of acute illness than do younger persons. Clearly, the older aged are a group in need of specialized services.

As this subgroup continues to increase, numerous approaches will be required to enable the over 75s to retain their independence as community members. It is in the best interest of both the older person and the community to assist such individuals in avoiding costly and debilitating institutional care. Many service models are presently being demonstrated in an effort to identify those approaches which respond best to the needs of the older elderly.

ENRICHED HOUSING PROGRAM

One of these approaches is specialized housing for the frail, which is often combined with a package of supportive services. This model has been in use now for many years in various forms and has emerged as a major approach to serving the frail.[1] The focus here will be on one such program, The Enriched Housing Program of the New York State Department of Social Services and, in particular,

The author wishes to thank Thelma Stackhouse, Central Office Administrator of the CSS Enriched Housing Program, for her help in preparing this chapter.

257

on the model employed at the Throgs Neck site in the Bronx, operated by The Community Service Society of New York. While this site serves an urban elderly population, the information gained from operation of this and other similar sites is valuable in meeting the needs of the frail in other settings.

Enriched Housing is a statewide program which combines some aspects of congregate living arrangements with a package of supportive services. The goal of the program is to provide a noninstitutional supportive living environment for functionally impaired individuals aged 65 and over allowing them to maintain an independent lifestyle. The program is operated by New York State through contracts with voluntary agencies for the administration of the individual sites. The service package includes a daily congregate meal, housekeeping services, heavy cleaning as needed, transportation and shopping assistance, information and referral services and counseling. Beyond this format each program varies according to the site and may include individual apartments (as is the case at the Throgs Neck site) or a large congregate living space with either single or shared rooms.

Funding for the program comes from three major sources. Start-up grants are provided by New York State to the contracting agency for purposes of obtaining space, hiring staff and purchasing furniture and equipment. Ongoing income is provided for SSI eligible individuals through the Congregate Level II support payment which the State has extended to residents of the program. This support payment is larger than the regular SSI payment amount and previously was available only to residents of Domiciliary Care Facilities. Those who are not SSI eligible pay a flat fee for the service package plus the monthly rent. In the case of the Throgs Neck site, rent is determined according to the income guidelines of the New York City Housing authority. The total space or group of apartments is rented by the sponsoring agency. The residents pay their rent plus the service package charge to the program or, in the case of SSI residents, their check is turned over to the program and the resident receives back a monthly allowance for personal needs. [At the start of the program this was $70 per month for residents of the Throgs Neck program.]

The Throgs Neck site was opened in January, 1979 at the Randal Balcom Houses of the New York City Housing Authority. The selection of a public housing site for the aged represented both a logical and necessary choice for the program, combining proximity to other older persons and a senior center with adequate, low rental housing which only public or publicly subsidized housing can provide. The site is located in an area isolated from shopping and transportation resources, however, and this has created problems which, while familiar to program directors in suburban or rural settings, are unusual for an urban setting.

The site consists of 18 apartments located in two clusters in adjoining buildings. Program guidelines specify that "only a small portion of units in any one building or apartment complex can be devoted to Enriched Housing in order to preserve a noninstitutional environment." While the intent of this guideline is laudable, the same effect might have been achieved by locating the apartment clusters on two floors of the same building. Such an arrangement might have allowed for more efficient management with a smaller staff.

Resident Characteristics—Reasons for Entering the Program

The program is open to persons 65 or over who are functionally impaired and unable to live independently without supports yet who neither require continuous nursing or other medical care nor full-time personal care. The planners originally expected that residents would span the entire over 65 age range, thus providing a mix of older and younger aged. The experience of the program has shown that this was an unrealistic expectation. Those younger aged who have applied have been, for the most part, too disabled to qualify for the program. Thus, during the first two years of operation, the program residents' age ranged between 70 and 83 with a median age of 76. Women have far outnumbered men (16 females to 4 males in the first two years operation of the Throgs Neck site) reflecting their greater numbers in this age group.

Those who have applied to the program have named inadequate housing most often as their immediate reason for so doing. Affordable housing, adequate to meet the needs of older functionally impaired persons, especially those who live alone, is in chronic shortage in the inner city neighborhoods of New York City and other urban areas of the United States. Projections indicate that the need for such housing will increase rapidly during the next 15 to 20 years.[2]

The immediate housing environment is often the most crucial factor in determining whether an older person can retain an independent lifestyle. Most older elderly spend more time in their home or apartment than anywhere else. The immediate household environment often poses little or no problem for the younger aged. However, a sudden change in mobility due to arthritis, stroke or other debilitating illness can easily cause a previously adequate housing environment to become intolerable. Many have tended to overlook the extent to which deteriorating health has contributed to the need for Enriched Housing and similar programs. Residents often cite housing as the reason for applying to the program when vision and hearing problems were actually heavy factors. A six room apartment may, overnight become too large to keep clean or negotiate easily. The absence of an elevator in a walk-up building can render an apartment unsuitable for a stroke victim or someone with severe hypertension or heart disease. These examples are illustrations of a problem faced by the older elderly every day—namely, how to remain as independent, autonomous individuals during a period of fixed income and declining functional ability. For many, services provided by a home care agency may be the answer. This is especially true for those with natural supports—friends and relatives—to look after them. However, there are others for whom congregate housing provides a "better fit."[3] The experience of the Throgs Neck Enriched Housing site is instructive.

The majority of those in the program either have no family immediately near them or did not wish to live with them. Enriched Housing has provided these individuals with another option to receive the care they need while allowing them to maintain an autonomy which is extremely important to persons in danger of institutionalization. Certainly, with the changing definition of family and household during the past few years, many types of living arrangements will be necessary to accommodate, in old age, the growing number of single persons, divorced and childless couples and others who did not fit into the standard two parent, two child household model.

Health Needs and Enriched Housing

During the first two years of the program, two residents died and two others were relocated to a more appropriate level of care when their health deteriorated. While more turnover has occurred than the planners had expected, this is not at all unusual for a population of older aged individuals.

The difficulty arises when a resident suffers an episode of acute illness. Experience indicates that this older population experiences periods of ill health which may not alter the overall long-term health care status but do require more intensive care, during these occurrences, than the program is designed to provide.

The challenge of a program such as this is to provide appropriate care to individuals whose health status may fluctuate, at reasonable cost and with a minimum of trauma for the resident. In the case of Enriched Housing, this has, at times, created difficulties for both the resident and the sponsoring agency. When a resident requires hospitalization, the sponsor's responsibility for the rent continues, even though residents on SSI have their grant reduced after a 30 day period of hospitalization. This policy deprives the program of vital income and is not consonant with what we know about the functioning of the older elderly. Such individuals do recover from serious periods of acute illness, but the process may often take more time for an older elderly individual. An understanding of this aspect of the care of the aged is needed in shaping public policy.

A strong case can be made that programs such as Enriched Housing fill a gap between unassisted community living and institutional care in a cost effective manner. Although the Throgs Neck site has made excellent use of networking and has many arrangements with other community services including hospitals and nursing homes, one major question is whether such a program might better be operated by a skilled nursing facility. Movement of individuals back and forth between levels of care might be easier under such arrangements. Additional nursing and/or other medical care might also be provided to a resident in their own apartment or room for short periods, especially if the program were located in reasonable proximity to a skilled nursing facility, thus allowing personnel to be deployed from one facility to another. There are, however, some serious drawbacks to such an arrangement. The task of maintaining the appropriate level of supportive services to meet the needs of the residents while at the same time retaining a noninstitutional environment is perhaps the most difficult challenge confronting the administrator. While close association with an SNF would certainly have administrative advantages, the closer one comes to the medical model, the more danger there is of crossing over the fine line which separates the institution from the noninstitutional program.

The Director—Necessary Skills

Those who manage and direct programs such as the Enriched Housing model require a variety of skills. This is true because enriched housing is more than a housing program and encompasses many services and delivery systems as a whole—transportation, social service, health care, meals, etc.

First and foremost a director of such a program must have the skills needed of any administrator. He or she must be skilled in supervision, budgeting and planning and will need good speaking and writing abilities. Other required skills are drawn from the traditional social work disciplines of casework, group work and community organization and planning. The director must wear many hats for the viability of the program depends on the provision of a wide range of services with a minimum of staff.

The individual older person residing in the enriched housing will demand certain casework skills of the director. Counseling, empathy, advocacy, knowledge of the larger service network and negotiating ability are needed. The residents spend time not only as individuals needing individually tailored casework help but frequently come together as a group. A director will be called upon to utilize group skills to an extent unknown by group workers in other situations. This is because special problems can arise in these circumstances in which the group members did not choose each other but came together through having applied and been accepted into the housing program. The director will need a thorough understanding of group dynamics, especially those related to how the group deals with the stress of losing members through death or transfer to a higher level of care, and acceptance of new members by a group which may have become cohesive with a high level of interaction over a period of time.

No service program can operate effectively without interaction with the surrounding community. Thus community organizing skills will be called upon. The ability to relate to politicians and government agencies as an advocate for individuals within the enriched housing program is needed. A good working relationship with the owner of the housing, whether private or public, is clearly essential as there will inevitably be policy and programming differences to resolve. The director must also be able to build a network of services to be called upon when needed. This takes time, patience and the ability to know and be known by the program directors of agencies, medical and nonmedical, in the service area.

In addition to a high level of skill in the traditional social work areas, an enriched housing director needs other skills and bodies of knowledge which usually fall outside a social worker's purview. The housing program is also a meals program and the director must understand the varied nutritional requirements of the residents and be able to plan menus which meet these needs. Food purchasing and food preparation skills are important. The health of residents is of primary concern and here the director needs knowledge of the many chronic and acute illnesses which can afflict the elderly. A basic understanding of symptomatology, emergency medical procedures and of pharmacology is helpful.

It is clear that the position of enriched housing director calls for a person with some working experience as well as a person with some special characteristics. Strengths to be looked for in a director are patience, unflappability, empathy, perseverance and the ability to integrate varied skills and knowledge areas towards developing a safe and inviting living environment for a community of frail elderly persons.

The Enriched Housing Program provides its residents with the opportunity to live for a longer period of time as independent individuals in a residential environment closely approximating that in which they have lived. More such programs must be developed if we are to meet the needs of the older elderly population. Financing must be available to help organizations with low capital reserves to set up and maintain programs. In the absence of adequate funding, many populations (minority groups come most quickly to mind) are deprived of the ability to sponsor and operate vitally needed programs in their communities. The turnover in the resident population, with the accompanying loss of income and cash flow problems, tends to limit sponsorship of housing type programs to large well-financed agencies which can accommodate such irregularities in income. This could create a barrier to widespread replication of the Enriched Housing model in New York State and elsewhere.

With a dependable source of financing, smoother procedures for moving individuals between levels of care, and with highly motivated and skilled staff, the model of assisted housing for the aged developed by New York State can make a significant contribution to the quality of life of the older elderly in the community.

REFERENCES

1. See Donahue, W. T., Thompson, M. M. & Curran, D. (Eds.). *Congregate Housing for Older People.* DHEW Publication No. (OHD) 77-20284, USGPO, Washington, D.C., 1977.

2. International Center for Social Gerontology. *Report on Congregate Housing.* Washington, D.C., 1978.

3. For further reading on the housing needs of the aged the reader is referred to the works of M. Powell Lawton, Wilma Donahue, Frances Carp and Leon Pastelan.

Author Index

A

Achenbaum, W.A. 28,34
Ackerman, N.A. 55,67
Adams, M. 108,119
Aikshe, H. 180
Aleichem, S. 245
Allan, C. 118
Allport, G.W. 5,11
Anderson, O. 137
Anglin, B. 105,119
Apter, D. 32
Arluck, F. 241-242
Armstron, H.F. 118
Arnhoff 125
Asch, C. 166
Atchley, R.C. 67

B

Bailey, M. 180
Baker, B.L. 113,118,119
Baron, S. 190
Barr, E. 221
Baxter, E. 137,139
Beaver, M.L. 54
Becker, E. 6,9,11
Becker, H. 138
Beckett, S. 243-244
Begab, M.J. 112,119
Beigel, A. 138
Bell, A. 119
Bell, D. 23
Bengtson, V.L. 61,96
Berezin, M. 137
Berger, P.L. 4,11
Berger, R.M. 82
Bergman, M. 191
Bettelheim, B. 191
Binstock, R. 34
Birren, J. 46,53
Black, K.D. 96
Blatt, B. 138
Blenkner, M. 59,68,78,81,82,83
Block, M.R. 82
Bloom, J. 228,229,242-243
Bloom, M. 79,81,82,83

Blum, A. 83
Boggs, E.M. 114,119
Boszormenyi-Nagy, I. 57,68
Brody, E. 68
Brotman, H. 38,39,40,42,44,53,118
Bruininks, R.H. 103-104,118
Burchinal, L. 11
Bush, G. 190
Busse, E. 139
Butler, R.N. 6,10,11,12,20,44,53,126,
130,139,140,151,210,243

C

Cahn, L. 150
Cain, L. 39,53
Calenbrander, A. 156,167
Callison, D.A. 105,118
Calvert, W.R. 95
Camus, A. 226
Cannon, R.L. 118
Cantor, M. 11
Carp, F. 264
Carter, R. 238
Caudill, W. 138
Chiovaro, S.J. 118
Clecak, P. 29,34
Cobbs, J. 255
Cole, T. 27,34
Coleridge, S.T. 225-226
Comfort, A. 68
Conot, R.E. 190
Coward, R.T. 96
Crystal, S. 15,33
Cummings, E. 138,139
Cummings, J. 138,139
Curran, D. 264

D

Danis, B. 68
Daum, M. 11,33,191
Davidson, S. 218,223
Davidson, W.S. 95
Davon, S. 255
Dawidowicz, L. 190
Des Pres, T. 139

J

Jackson, J.J. 44,53,87,95
Jacobs, B. 24,34
Jacobskind, B. 141,144
Janowitz, M. 33
Jarvik, L.F. 119
Jenkins, S. 95
Johnsen, P. 68
Jucovy, M. 191
Jung, C.J. 10,12
Justice, R.S. 102,118

K

Kalish, R.A. 21,33
Kaminsky, M. 141,146,151,191,210
Kane, Rbt. 137,138,139
Kane, R. 137,138
Kelleher, D.K. 165,168
Kimmel, D. 151
King, A. 33
Kirschbaum, D. 221,222
Kirschner, C. 68
Kirchner, C. 157-158,167
Koestler, F.A. 166,167
Komorovsky, M. 255
Kornblum, S. 222
Kosberg, J.I. 82,83
Kramer, M. 139
Krill, D. 68
Krystal, H. 191
Kubie, S.H. 210
Kudla, M.J. 118
Kumbar 125
Kushler, M.G. 95
Kutza, E. 34

L

Ladd, E. 33
Laird, C. 137,138
Lakin, K.C. 103-104,118
Landau, G. 210
Lau, E.E. 82,83
Lawrence 139
Lawton, M.P. 7,11,138,264
Lazarus 126,139
Lehmann, V. 81
Lesser, J. 140
Levenson, A. 138
Levi, P. 191
Levin, S. 214,222
Levine, E. 139
Levison, A. 255
Lewis, M. 6,11,53,126,130,139,140,
   151,210,243
Lichtheim, G. 33

Lifton, R.J. 191
Lindey, E. 81
Linzer, N. 191
Lipset, S. 23
Lipsett, B. 229,240
Lipstadt, D. 190
Litwak, E. 87,95,137,140,223
Long, M. 164,168
Love, J. 163,167
Lowman, C. 157-158,167
Lowy, L. 118
Luckmann, T. 4,11
Lukoff, I.F. 166
Lynes, J.K. 81

M

MacLeod, T. 222
Maddox, G. 138
Mahoney, S.C. 110,119
Marsden, C.D. 139
Marx, K. 33
Mathiasen, G. 81
Mayer, M. 180
McAdam, D. 33
McCarthy, T. 34
McCaslin, R. 95
McConnell, S.R. 39,53
McLaughlin, J.S. 82
Mellor, M.J. 68
Mendelson, M. 138
Mendenhall 125
Mercer, J. 118
Merriam, S. 140
Meyer, J. 34
Meyerhoff, B. 10,12,210
Miller, S.J. 67
Minuchin, S. 68
Monk, A. 67,118,180
Montale, E. 225-226
Moody, H.R. 235,244
Moroney, R. 138,140
Morrison, B. 95

N

Napier, A.Y. 68
Neugarten, B.L. 25,34,39,53,69,138
Neuman, F. 104,106,118,119
Nickell, J.P. 82
Niederland, W. 191
Nielsen, M.A. 79,81,82,83
Nirje, B. 119

O

O'Brien, B. 222
O'Connell, P. 68
O'Connor, G. 102,118

Subject Index